Disclaimer & Copyright

Text Copyright © Siim Land 2016

All rights reserved. No part of this guide may be reproduced in any form without permission in writing from the publisher except in the case of brief quotations embodied in critical articles or reviews.

Legal & Disclaimer

The information contained in this book is not designed to replace or take the place of any form of medicine or professional medical advice. The information in this book has been provided for educational and entertainment purposes only.

The information contained in this book has been compiled from sources deemed reliable, and it is accurate to the best of the Author's knowledge; however, the Author cannot guarantee its accuracy and validity and cannot be held liable for any errors or omissions. Changes are periodically made to this book. You must consult your doctor or get professional medical advice before using any of the suggested remedies, techniques, or information in this book.

Upon using the information contained in this book, you agree to hold harmless the Author from and against any damages, costs, and expenses, including any legal fees potentially resulting from the application of any of the information provided by this guide. This disclaimer applies to any damages or injury caused by the use and application, whether directly or indirectly, of any advice or information presented, whether for breach of contract, tort, negligence, personal injury, criminal intent, or under any other cause of action.

You agree to accept all risks of using the information presented inside this book. You need to consult a professional medical practitioner in order to ensure you are both able and healthy enough to participate in this program.

All rights reserved. No part of this publication may be reproduced, distributed, or transmitted in any form or by any means, including photocopying, recording, or other electronic or mechanical methods, without the prior written permission of the publisher, except in the case of brief quotations embodied in critical reviews and certain other noncommercial uses permitted by copyright law. For permission requests, contact the publisher, at the address below.

http://www.siimland.com.

Cover design by Siim Land.

Table of Contents

Disclaimer & Copyright 1

Table of Contents 4

Introduction A Scene from the Matrix 10

Chapter I 101 Time with Ketosis and your Body 16

    Indigenous Ketogenic Societies 21

    Is Ketosis Safe 23

Chapter II Why do a Ketogenic Diet…At Least Once 27

    Ketosis for Health 29

    Athletes Going Against the Grain 31

    Keto Smart 34

    Sleep Like the Sleeping Beauty 36

Chapter III How to Get into the Exclusive Keto Club 39

The Big Fat Lies and Myths Debunked 40

Get into Ketosis 43

    Carbohydrates 45

    Protein 51

    Fats 55

Symptoms of Withdrawal 62

Am I in Ketosis? 63

    Water weight loss 66

    You're thirsty 66

    Keto breath 67

    Metallic taste in your mouth 68

    Stinky urine 68

    Slight headaches and fatigue 68

    Lack of appetite 69

    After Adaptation 69

Do I Have to be in Ketosis? 71

Chapter IV To Get Fat Adapted Don't Do This. 73

Too Many Carbs to Adapt 73

How to Read Nutrition Labels 75

Too Much Protein, Bro 79

Not Enough Fat…What? 81

Additional Factors 82

Chapter V Intermittent Fasting 87

Chapter VI A Definitive Guide to Starting the Ketogenic Diet 97

It Starts with a Healthy Gut 99

What Changes You Should Make 102

Keto Shopping List 109

Superfoods 123

Chapter VII The Ketogenic Cookbook 127

The Ultimate Breakfast 127

Fatty Egg Yolk Coffee 129

Bone Broth Soup 132

Meaty Vegetable Roast-Feast 135

Kale Chips 137

Cauliflower Pizza 139

Cheesy Tomato Soup 142

Bacon and Egg Muffins 144

Coconut Cream Porridge 147

Bacon Brussel Sprouts 148

Pan Fried Avocado 150

Breakfast Tacos 151

Coconut Keto Cereal 153

Bacon Bread 155

Cauli Hash 157

Avocado Mayonnaise 159

Beef Stroganoff	162
Keto Spaghetti Squash	164
Cheesy Grated Cauliflower	166
Keto Sushi	168
Coconut Milk Ice Cream	170
Keto Pancakes	172
Keto Chocolate	175
Chocolate Peanut Butter Fat Bomb Cups	177
Vanilla Ice Cream	179
Keto Brownies	180
How Should You Eat?	183
Chapter VIII Simple Keto Supplements	186
Not Really Supplements	189
Supplements you HAVE to Take	192
Supplements Empowered	194

Bonus Chapter How to Get into Ketosis Super Fast 201

    How to Get Into Ketosis Fast 202

    Mistakes to Avoid 204

Conclusion Beyond Burning Fat and Ketosis 206

Ultimate Keto Meal Plan 209

More Books from the Author 210

Leave a Review on Amazon! 214

About the Author. 215

References 217

Introduction
A Scene from the Matrix

Decades have passed since the food industry and medical community started to villainize fat. Together with its brother in arms, cholesterol, they turned into mythical entities who had released the obesity epidemic onto the world. For some mysterious reason, people couldn't tolerate red meat, butter, bacon and cheese anymore, even though they had been a part of the aboriginal menu in all parts of the world.

The opposite became the norm. Whole grain cereals, breads whiter than snow, diet yogurts, chicken thinner than air, skimmed milk... zero fat everything! This seemed to solve the issue, but they were oh so wrong. The jaws of the food industry started spewing out high fructose corn syrup, monosodium glutamate and hydrogenated trans fats as if it was the river Nile. As the meat got leaner and food lower in calories, the population became even more obese and diseased. What gives?

Luckily, thanks to the resurgence of the ancestral living movement and the Paleo community, we've come back full circle to the nutrition our body actually yearns for. Of course, it's not the magical answer we've been searching for, but what scientific research and biohacking shows us is that we're heading in the right direction. At least for the time being.

You have probably picked up this book for a similar reason. The ketogenic diet has become widely popular and has proven to be extremely effective. Not only for weight loss, but for battling diabetes as well. For me, the greatest benefits go far beyond that. I don't suffer from any medical condition nor carry any excess weight. To be honest, getting any leaner than I currently am wouldn't be healthy. I eat keto, not because of the effortless year-round single-digit body fat percentage, but because of the utter sense of enjoyment I get. My name is Siim Land and after having followed a ketogenic diet for a long time, I must say that I've never felt better.

That's why I decided to write this book as well. Ketosis is an amazing tool to use but for the inexperienced practitioner it may turn into a nightmare. If you don't have much knowledge about low carb eating, then consider yourself very lucky. As the title suggests, I'm going to teach you Simple Keto, a way to start a ketogenic diet, without losing your mind, stressing out or damaging your health in the process. Einstein's infamous quote illustrates my point perfectly: *"Everything should be made as simple as possible. But not simpler."* It's not rocket science, but it's still science, Einstein...

This is not just another low carb book nor is it a diet program. In addition to that, it's also a source of invaluable knowledge you need to live a healthy lifestyle. **Between these pages lies the STRONGER, SMARTER, LEANER, HEALTHIER and HAPPIER version of yourself.** By making the right decisions and implementing the plan correctly, you'll be able to get into ketosis in no time. This can be as life transforming for you as it has been for me. Hopefully you have enough guts to carry through.

Here's what you'll get from Simple Keto.

- Burn body fat, not muscle. Weight loss doesn't equal fat loss.

- Improve your mental focus and make your mind as sharp as a knife.
- Battle diabetes and potentially reverse it.
- Improve your health markers, such as blood pressure, blood sugar levels, cholesterol etc.
- Protect yourself against cancer, tumors and coronary heart disease.
- Increase your longevity and insulin sensitivity.
- Become fat adapted and start using fat for fuel.
- Experience mental clarity and feel amazing.
- Have access to abundant energy all the time.
- Reduce your hunger and lose sugar cravings for good.
- Eat mouthwatering and delicious meals that leave you satiated for long periods of time.

These nutrition wars resemble The Matrix. Most of the population is asleep and plugged into the system. A few are awake and know what lies beneath the veil.

I'm not saying that keto is the end-all-be-all. It's just that the standard American diet (SAD - I know, right?) has caused too much damage that now needs to be reversed. Going low carb is just a very effective way of doing it.

Right now you're faced with the same question as Neo was. Take the blue pill and you fall back asleep. You'll wake up like nothing ever happened. Take the red pill and I'll show you how deep the rabbit hole really goes.

Chapter I
101 Time with Ketosis and your Body

Let's get right to it and keep it simple stupid. We have to start from the beginning and go through some of the fundamentals of keto. There's going to be some science, but don't worry I could even explain it to a child.

There are different fuel sources the body uses. When we're born, we get all of the energy we need from our mother's breast milk, at least that's what we did in the past, which puts us into ketosis. As we grow up, we begin to eat different foods, comprising of the 3 macronutrients: protein, carbs and fat. This primes our body to be using glucose, which is a carbohydrate molecule, and sets it as our primary default fuel source. There's nothing wrong with that, the thing is that in today's society most people have drifted too far away from their aboriginal ketogenic pathways, which causes obesity, diabetes and other ailments. Luckily, there is a way to circumvent that.

The human body is a complex system that can adapt to almost anything. It has found a solution to solving the bioenergetics component of being self-sufficient and resourceful. Ketosis is just that – an irreplaceable part of our biology that creates endogenous (from within) energy.

In a nutshell, ketosis is a metabolic state in which the body has shifted from using glucose as the primary fuel source into supplying its energy demands with ketone bodies. This happens when the liver glycogen stores are depleted and a substitute is necessary for the brain to maintain its functioning.

Both carbohydrates and fats can be used for the production of energy, but they're different in quality. However, in the presence of both, the body will always prefer carbs because sugar can be easily accessed and quickly absorbed. To get the most out of the ketones and fatty acids, there needs to be a period of keto-adaptation. The length of it depends on how reliant you are of glucose and how well your body accepts this new fuel source.

Ketosis is an altered, but still natural, metabolic state that occurs either over a prolonged period of fasting or by restricting carbohydrate intake significantly, usually up to less than 50 grams per day [i]**.**

After an overnight fast already, our liver glycogen stores will be depleted and *Captain Liver* starts to produce more ketone bodies. This, in return, will increase the availability of fatty acids in the blood stream which the body then begins to utilize for the production of energy. It can be derived from both food and the adipose tissue.

This process is called beta-oxidation. When fat is broken down by the liver, glycerol and fatty acid molecules are released. The fatty acid gets broken down even more through ketogenesis that produces a ketone body called acetoacetate. This is then converted further into two other type of ketone bodies. (1) Beta-hydroxybutyrate (BHB), which is the preferred fuel source for the brain and (2) acetone, that can be metabolized into glucose, but is mainly excreted as waste.

When you're running on glucose you go down the pathway of glycolysis and create pyruvate. All of these actions get burned inside the mitochondria and you can get <u>25% more energy from using beta-hydroxybutyrate</u> as fuel. In this scenario of fat utilization, we're taking the more efficient route that increases the density of our cellular power plants.

Achieving the Optimal Fat Burning State

- Sugar Burner
- Fat Storing
- Ketosis (Goodbye Carb Cravings)
- Nutritional Ketosis (Fat Burning Machine)
- Fat Burning

Nutritional ketosis is not the same as ketoacidosis, which causes the pH levels in the blood to drop and become acidic. This can result with a coma and eventually death. Usually, the body manages to maintain the acidity of the blood within a normal range despite the presence of ketones. Ketoacidosis occurs mostly with type-1 diabetes and excessive alcohol consumption.

The shift from burning sugar and becoming fat adapted causes a lot of changes in your physiology. After the initial period of adaptation, the body's biochemistry will be completely altered.

Approximately 75% of the energy used by the brain will be provided by ketones and the liver will change its enzymes from dominantly digesting carbohydrates to actually preferring fat [ii]. Protein catabolism decreases significantly, as fat stores are mobilized and the use of ketones increases. Muscle glycogen gets used even less and the majority of our caloric demands will be derived from the adipose tissue.

Nutritional ketosis is perfectly safe and a great metabolic state to be in. This process is an adaptive response and completely normal. During periods of famine it will enable us to survive and maintain our vitality. If we the body doesn't know how to use its stored fat for fuel, it would perish, once it runs out of sugar.

Indigenous Ketogenic Societies

Over the course of history, most aboriginal tribes have subsisted solely on high fat diets. In environments where there aren't many plants to be found, people rely primarily on meat.

The Innuit and Eskimos have lived off whale blubber, seal meat, salmon, cheese and caribou meat for centuries. Fat is their most precious commodity, as it gives them the extra calories they need to survive in such harsh climate. In fact, rent on land in some places is paid with butter. Despite that high amount of saturated fat and cholesterol in their diet, heart disease, diabetes and cancer were largely unknown. Only after they came in contact with white man's white refined carbohydrates did other diseases of the civilization catch up with them and they got obese.

The Masai tribe in Africa also follows a ketogenic diet. They're pastoralists and subsist mainly on their cattle, by eating their meat, drinking their unpasteurized milk and raw milk. Masai warriors are definitely a lot healthier and fitter than the majority of the people in our society.

Even in the Western world there are nations who eat a ton of fat. The Mediterranean Diet is thought to be the healthiest of them all. It consists of mainly fish, olive oil, cheese and vegetables. People from this region have less heart disease and better blood markers. Researchers from the States figured that it had to do with the low amount of saturated fat and cholesterol in their food. However, the Greek Orthodox Church also preaches a lot of fasting, which has even more profound health benefits. In fact, the more religious folk fast more than 200 days a year. This is the real cause for their vitality. As this ancient healing practice gets less popular amongst young people, disease begins to rise again because there are still a lot of refined grains and carbohydrates in the diet.

Is Ketosis Safe

One fear that ordinary physicians have about the ketogenic diet is that it can't sustain healthy functioning of an organism. Apart from developing ketoacidosis you'll also starve to death, which is false. How will your body and brain survive if there are no carbohydrates?

An essential nutrient is something that's required for normal physiological functioning and the survival of the organism[iii]. It cannot be synthesized by the body and thus has to be obtained from a dietary source. Carbohydrates are non-essential, unlike amino acids and fatty acids, which we don't actually need to live and can function very well without.

Amino acids and fat are essential building blocks of all the cells in our body. Protein is used to create new muscle tissue, whereas the lipids balance our hormones that instigate these processes in the first place and protect cell membrane.

The biggest reason why we have to consume so many calories every single day is to feed our hungry brain. It comprises less than 5% of our body weight but demands about 20% of our total energy expenditure. To maintain stable blood sugar levels and a caloric balance, it needs to have access to fuel all of the time.

The brain can use only about 120 grams of glucose a day [iv], which means you still need at least 30 grams of glucose while running on max ketones. That doesn't mean it ought to come from dietary carbohydrates.

During a process called *gluconeogenesis* (creation of new sugar), the liver converts amino acids found in food and glycerol, which is the backbone of triglycerides, into glucose. While in a deep fasted state, glycerol can contribute up to 21.6% of glucose production [v]. It's estimated that about 200 grams of glucose can be manufactured daily by the liver and kidneys from dietary protein and fat intake [vi].

Once you keto-adapt, your body and brain won't even need that much glucose, as they will happily use ketones instead. Carbohydrates are the default fuel source but not because they're better than fatty acids by any means. The body simply prefers it because it's easy to store and quick to absorb.

However, the brain is made up of 60% fat and runs a lot better on ketones. In fact, the high amounts of fat found in animal products and meat were probably one of the driving forces of our increased brain size. According to the Expansive Tissue Hypothesis posed by the anthropologists Leslie Aiello and Peter Wheeler suggests that the metabolic requirements of large brains were offset by a corresponding reduction of the gut[vii]. As our stomachs got smaller, our neocortices got larger. By eating solely plant foods, we wouldn't have managed to get enough excess energy for our neural network to improve itself.

In ketosis, the brain begins to use less glucose and the small amount it needs can be derived from ketogenic foods. Muscles begin to release less glycogen as well and the entire body starts using ketones for fuel. It makes the entire organism more efficient and powerful.

Chapter II

Why do a Ketogenic Diet...At Least Once

But why should we want to enter ketosis when food is abundant. Hopefully, you're beginning to see the slowly emerging advantages of this already. In comparison to the contemporary approach, the ketogenic diet looks very appealing. There are a lot of health benefits to this, covering both physical and mental aspects.

The most obvious advantage is increased fat oxidation[viii]. By consuming carbohydrates our body will secrete more insulin. When this hormone is elevated we're more prone to storing rather than burning fat. If it's constantly high, we'll never be able to actually tap into using our own resources. This is beneficial not only for a lean physique but, most importantly, to teach the body these vital pathways.

Abundance of food will already prevent famine and some people don't even enter a fasted state, ever. In this scenario, I would imagine, utilizing our own adipose tissue would eventually become foreign to us. The consequences to that are self-explanatory and detrimental. We're not faced with starvation and have circumvented hunger but we can't expect things to stay the same forever.

When you're running on glucose you go down the pathway of glycolysis and create pyruvate. All of these actions get burned inside the mitochondria and you can get <u>25% more energy</u> from using beta-hydroxybutyrate as fuel. In this scenario of fat utilization, we're taking the more efficient route that increases the density of our cellular power plants.

The by-products of glucose metabolism are advanced glycation end-products (AGEs), which promote inflammation and oxidative stress[ixx], by binding a protein or lipid molecule with sugar. They speed up aging[xi], and can cause diabetes. This doesn't happen when burning clean fuel - quality fat. Also, the constantly elevated levels of circulating blood sugar are associated with nerve malfunctioning, high morbidity, bacterial infection, cancer progression and Alzheimer's.

The #1 food for tumors is sugar.

Ketosis reduces natural hunger to a bare minimum and regulates appetite[xii]. This is the result of the body being able to generate energy from both the adipose tissue and dietary fat intake. The ability to go without meals for 24 hours while not suffering any stomach pains or carb driven cravings of insanity is incredibly empowering, not to mention useful.

Our body is made to burn fat. The adipose tissue is like a black hole with infinite storage capacity. Any surplus calorie we don't need right away gets deposited for future use. When in ketosis, we'll be withdrawing energy from our own body fat to maintain a caloric balance.

Ketones are the "superfuel" above both glucose and free fatty acids.

Ketosis for Health

Because of the fact that a fat molecule has twice the amount of calories than a carbohydrate it gets digested a lot slower. **Unlike sugar, that gets burned up easily, ketones move steadily and provide long lasting energy.**

This also prevents any rise in blood sugar from taking place, which happens after consuming something with a high glycemic index. Instant bursts of energy will inevitably fall as quickly. What goes up must come down. This results in hypoglycemia (a crash of blood sugar) and sleepiness. With fat that doesn't happen as we will have an abundant fuel source thus always feeling great. Instead of secreting insulin and taking our bodies for a rollercoaster ride we maintain a steady stream.

Following a low carbohydrate high fat diet has been proven very effective against a lot of the chronic illnesses people struggle with.

- Reduction in triglycerides[xiii]

- Increase in HDL cholesterol (the good one)[xiv]

- Drop in blood pressure[xv] and insulin levels[xvi]

All of which prevent heart disease, diabetes and metabolic syndrome[xvii]. For optimal health it looks very appealing.

Mark my words when I say that ketosis will help to cure cancer in the near future, as it's already being used as effective treatment. At the moment science is just beginning to fully understand and utilize this metabolic pathway.

Athletes Going Against the Grain

Another benefit is that in ketosis we will always have a lot of energy readily available. The maximum amount of glucose our bodies can store is about 2000 calories (approximately 400 grams of carbohydrates in the muscles and 100 grams in the liver.) Once this runs out then more fatty acids are produced to supply the demand. Although this is the point in which adipose tissue is being used it only happens to a certain extent. To still get some form of glucose the body will also begin to break down a bit of the protein in muscles and organs to produce sugar. The reason for doing so is because it's not that adapted to primarily using ketones. To prevent that from happening a person would need to be constantly adding in more carbohydrates to fuel their activities.

In ketosis, however, the main source of energy is significantly bigger. **Even the leanest of people with 7% body fat carry around at least 20 000 worth of calories with them at all times on their own bodies.** Refeeding isn't necessary as there is always some fuel available. This also preserves muscles and other vital organs from being catabolized. Instead of being a quick sugar burner we can become efficient fat burners instead.

Stored calories.   7%   10%

20 000 -30 000 calories

Ketogenic dieting is becoming very popular amongst endurance athletes, especially ultra-runners and ironman triathletes who have to perform at a high level for extreme durations. By carrying around their own fuel on their bodies they can tap into an abundance of energy. They literally go against the grain of everything in optimal sport's nutrition.

For instance, Sami Inkinen and his wife, Meredith Loring rowed across the Pacific Ocean from California to Hawaii in 45 days while following a low-carb sugar-free high-fat ketogenic diet. Despite being physically active for 21 hours a day they did not suffer any decrease in performance, health or cravings for carbs. Such adaptation shows that we are capable of a lot more than we actually think. How else did our ancestors complete their epic journeys of exploration and migration?

In a study on advanced triathletes the group who followed a ketogenic approach instead of the traditional high-carb diet showed 2-3 times higher peak fat oxidation during submaximal exercise[xviii].

Contrary to popular belief physical performance does not suffer by ditching the carbs. It is also used in strength sports such as powerlifting and gymnastics[xix] where the intensities are lot higher. Bodybuilders also use periods of low-carb eating to prepare for shows and improve body composition.

In my own experience, I haven't noticed any negative side-effects of ketosis after proper adaptation. I have managed to improve every aspect of my training and health. It definitely feels great and is well worth the effort.

Keto Smart

In addition to performance oriented benefits ketosis also has cognitive and mental ones. There's a big difference between being high on ketones versus sugar.

Because of how evolutionarily valuable glucose is, the brain's reward system lights up every time we consume it making us want more. Cravings and hunger pains come from some people's mind kicking into overdrive and losing their reason over something sweet.

Sugar cravings are caused by an energy crisis in the body. If the brain doesn't get access to fuel it will try to motivate you to find something to eat. Because by default it only knows how to use glucose, it will also expect to have it.

However, if you're plugged into your largest fuel tank, your own body fat, then you won't experience these cravings. That's why people lose their sweet tooth completely when on a low carb diet. Their body detoxifies itself from sugar and the mind will get clearer.

Sugar doesn't actually provide us with that much energy and is mainly an illusion. It's a way of trapping our own ATP production. We might have a lot of stored calories but we won't be able to access them. That's why it's important to go through keto adaptation to teach the body how to use fat for fuel.

By avoiding carbohydrates, we also avoid the ups and downs of blood sugar, thus allowing our brain to function properly. By having a steady stream of energy it doesn't have to be on the lookout for glucose. Some is indeed needed which gets created by the liver but the majority can be derived from ketones. This type of eating has been used to cure children of epilepsy and is now being studied for other disorders as well, such as Alzheimer's and Parkinson's disease.

With the brain satisfied our cognition has the opportunity to flourish. This allows us to maintain mental clarity and avoid mind fog, which accompanies the consumption of whole grains. The majority of the brain is made up of fat, and the more you eat it, the better it can function.

We can think more clearly and with less disruption. Our ability to concentrate increases and I dare say that so does our intelligence. Who knows, maybe our IQ does so as well. Not directly, but as a result of being able to allocate our energy into appropriate channels and activities that make us smarter. Personally, I've definitely noticed a lot of improvement in this area.

Sleep Like the Sleeping Beauty

Additionally, the quality of our sleep improves because of the stability in blood sugar. If we run out of glucose in the middle of the night, then we will become hypoglycemic. Our starving brain will wake us up to get some fuel for survival. Midnight snacking is another example of people feeding all of the time and a bad habit to have.

Constant stream of energy means that there's no need to recharge as much, resulting in quality slumber. This way we can go through full sleep cycles and actually enter the deepest stages of recovery where all dreaming occurs and the magic happens. During my own periods of ketosis, I've gone through the entire night like a log without waking up.

What you will also see that you get less tired overall when on keto. Physical activities become less demanding and your endurance will increase. If you're obese, then you'll reclaim your enthusiasm and vitality towards life.

Once you go through the shift and eat appropriately, your body will heal itself. Inflammation disappears and you'll have less aches and pains. You may think that it's normal to be feeling this way now, but that's because you don't know that there's another way.

All of these benefits are the reason why you should try a ketogenic diet… at least once. It will give you high end physical as well as cognitive performance and is incredibly healthy.

Being in this metabolic state is very advantageous, as we become more resourceful with our own supplies and can thus always be excelling at whatever we're doing. You're going to have to keep it a secret, but the military is also very interested in this and is actively testing it on topnotch soldiers. When in ketosis we literally can become Superhuman.

Chapter III

How to Get into the Exclusive Keto Club

Nutritional ketosis goes against the grain (pun intended) and contradicts almost everything that is considered to be healthy nowadays. While the standard guidelines recommend about 50-60% of carbohydrates, ketogenic diets remain under 5%. Instead, what gets used the most is fat, making up to 70-80% of the macronutrient ratios. The blood pressure of some people probably went through the roof as they heard that. Because of decades of conditioning and brainwashing we have received it's natural to think this way.

	Total	Goal
■ Carbohydrates	6 %	5 %
■ Fat	73 %	80 %
▦ Protein	21 %	15 %

But isn't fat bad for our health? Definitely not. This fat-phobia is the result of false and biased science which based their results on studies with the wrong context.

<u>The Big Fat Lies and Myths Debunked</u>

Of course, fat is dangerous with elevated levels of insulin. During glycation sugar and fat molecules attach to each other, that create AGEs, and begin to circulate the blood stream for a longer period of time. This will cause oxidation and impairs the functioning of biomolecules. Doing this kills our mitochondria and causes cellular death. It also speeds up aging and will most definitely lead to disease.

Nutritional ketosis alters our metabolism completely and makes us use various fuel sources completely differently. **Keto adaptation increases the rate at which the body burns saturated fat for fuel and maintains better overall glucose levels.**

Fat in of itself is actually a lot better for us as it's vital for a lot of hormonal production and is more satiating. Saturated fat is needed for our neurotransmitters to work, making it essential for cognitive health and performance. We just must not mix it together with carbohydrates, ever.

The type of fat eaten is also important. In ketosis you're under different metabolic conditions than with a high carbohydrate diet. When fat is used for fuel, the body prefers more quality mono-unsaturates and saturates. As a sugar burner those things may not be as appealable.

The fatty parts of the animal are more nutritious and were valued most by hunter-gatherers. Indigenous people with unprocessed high meat diets were perfectly healthy, until they came in contact with the food industries of the West. The combination of their traditional way of eating and the introduction of refined carbohydrates resulted in disease, tooth decay and obesity[xx].

Another depicted villain is cholesterol which is produced by the body and needed for cell walls, bile production, vitamin D, brain and nerve functioning and hormonal production. It's an essential structural component of all animal cell membranes. Consumption of cholesterol does not increase it because of the feedback mechanism. There is no good or bad cholesterol, simply in a specific context it rises too high and becomes lethal.

One more fear is salt. Sodium intake necessary for human life especially on the ketogenic diet. Again, it's the wrong context that creates all of the problems and dangers. High carbohydrate intake makes the kidneys retain salt, whereas a low carb diet increases sodium exertion by the kidney (called the natriuresis of fasting).

Despite the ethical dilemma, eating meat is beneficial for us. Our intestinal track isn't designed to absorb cellulose. After our species adopted hunting we gained access to more calories. As a result of spending less time digesting food our gut decreased and brain size increased by allocating more energy to it. We got smarter not only because of the metabolic processes that ensued but also thanks to the way animals had to be hunted and meat cooked. Let's be honest here, it takes a lot more persistence, patience and cognition to hunt than to gather. However, fishing is even better than that. Making traps, harpoons and fish nets promotes ingenuity and social co-operation. Seafood and oily fish are rich in DHA, omega-3s which benefit our brain and health.

Get into Ketosis

The food on a ketogenic diet is mostly animal based. Most of the calories come from either meat, fish, eggs or other rich sources of fat such as butter. Despite the low allowance for carbohydrates it doesn't mean that no plants are consumed. Quite the contrary.

When you compare the amount of food in volume then vegetables make up the majority of the plate. They simply have that much less calories than fat but are bigger in size. So, it might seem almost like a vegetarian diet given how much fiber it provides. It's probably a lot more than the public dietary guidelines recommend, which is a good thing. Even some vegans might be surprised how much greens are actually eaten.

To induce ketosis insulin needs to be suppressed for an extended period of time. As a result, glucagon goes up and starts to empty the liver's glycogen stores. This is achieved by using our current storage and not eating high glycemic carbohydrates that raise our blood sugar even before we can put them into our mouth. Protein does so as well but to a much lesser degree and more steadily. Add fat into the mix and it will happen even more slowly. Leafy green vegetables are also safe as the actual amount of sugar in them is small in comparison to their fiber content, which decreases the rate of absorption.

Carbohydrates

Total caloric proportion is less than 5%. In total, the carbohydrate intake would be around 30 grams, fiber not included. The less of them, the faster will ketosis be induced.

Safe sources are fibrous leafy green and cruciferous vegetables, including other foods.

Food	Amount	Fat	NET Carbs (g)	Protein (g)
Lettuce, Butterhead	2oz/56 grams	0	0.5	1
Beet Greens	2oz/56 grams	0	0.5	1

Bok Choy	2oz/56 grams	0	0.5	1
Spinach	2oz/56 grams	0	1	1.5
Alfalfa Sprouts	2oz/56 grams	0	1	2
Swiss Chard	2oz/56 grams	0	1	1
Arugula	2oz/56 grams	0	1	1.5
Celery	2oz/56 grams	0	1	0.5

Lettuce	2oz/56 grams	0	1	0.5
Asparagus	2oz/56 grams	0	1	1
Eggplant	2oz/56 grams	0	1	0.5
Mushrooms, White	2oz/56 grams	0	1.5	2
Tomatoes	2oz/56 grams	0	1	0.5
Cauliflower	2oz/56 grams	0	1.5	1

Green Bell Pepper	2oz/56 grams	0	1.5	0.5
Cabbage	2oz/56 grams	0	2	1
Broccoli	2oz/56 grams	0	2	1.5
Green Beans	2oz/56 grams	0	2	1
Brussels Sprouts	2oz/56 grams	0	2.5	1.5
Kale	2oz/56 grams	0	2	2

Food	Amount	Fat (g)	NET Carbs (g)	Protein (g)
Artichoke	2oz/56 grams	0	2.5	2
Kelp	2oz/56 grams	0	3	1
Zucchini	2oz/56 grams	0	2	1

There are also a small variety of fruits and berries you can consume.

Food	Amount	Fat (g)	NET Carbs (g)	Protein (g)
Rhubarb	100 grams	0	2	1

Raspberries	100 grams	0	5	1.5
Blueberries	100 grams	0	10	2
Strawberries	100 grams	0	5	1
Blackberries	100 grams	0	5	1.5

Top 5 recommendations for carbohydrates are:

- Spinach
- Kelp
- Broccoli
- Cauliflower
- Cabbage

Protein

Total caloric proportion at about 15 %. Careful not to consume lean bits without any fat to slow down the absorption as it might get converted into sugar. The body will always try to find glucose. During the adaptation phase it will happen more easily than later. Pure protein with nothing else will go through glyconeogenesis (creation of new sugar). Best stick to fatty chunks.

Meat is obviously one of the best source.

Food	Amount	Fat (g)	NET Carbs (g)	Protein
Pork Chops	100 grams	14	0	24
Chicken Drumstick	1 medium drumstick	8	0	9

Chicken Wing	1 medium drumstick	7	0	8
Bacon	100 grams	42	0	37
Beef, Ground	100 grams	15	0	26
Lamb and Mutton	100 grams	21	0	25
Venison	100 grams	5	0	31
Liver, mammalian, fowl	100 grams	5	4	26

Duck	100 grams	28	0	19
Wild Boar	100 grams	4	0	28

Additionally, fatty fish, such as

Food	Amount	Fat (g)	NET Carbs (g)	Protein
Salmon	100 grams	13	0	20
Sardines	100 grams	13	0	25
Herring	100 grams	9	0	18
Mackerel	100 grams	25	0	19

Anchovies	100 grams	10	0	29
Sprats	100 grams	15	0	20

The best source of protein are probably eggs. They have the entire amino acid profile and are full of omega-3s, DHA, EPA and cholesterol, which is great for the cells and brain. Nutrition of 1 large egg: 5 grams of fat, 1 gram of carbs, 6 grams of protein.

However, some caution needs to be taken. All of those things can't be taken equally. Some pre-packaged products have added sugar in them and under many names (dextrose, glucose, fructose, maltodextrin, xylitol etc.) all of which ought to be avoided for best results.

Top 5 recommendations for protein are:

- Eggs
- Salmon

- Beef
- Pork
- Chicken

Fats

To be honest, there isn't actually a limit to how much fat we should be consuming. The more of it, the more ketones will be produced. With no carbohydrates in the menu we need to have another fuel source for the body.

In order to get into ketosis, we need to eat fat and a lot of it. What I'm talking about is adding it on our vegetables, protein, coffee - everywhere.

Food	Amount	Fat (g)	NET Carbs (g)	Protein
Butter	28 grams/1oz	28	0	0

Ghee	28 grams/1oz	28	0	0
Lard	28 grams/1oz	28	0	0
Tallow	28 grams/1oz	28	0	0
Avocado Oil	28 grams/1oz	28	0	0
Cocoa Butter	28 grams/1oz	28	0	0

Coconut Oil	28 grams/1oz	28	0	0
Flaxseed Oil	28 grams/1oz	28	0	0
Macadamia Oil	28 grams/1oz	28	0	0
MCT Oil	28 grams/1oz	28	0	0
Olive Oil	28 grams/1oz	28	0	0

Red Palm Oil	28 grams/1oz	28	0	0
Coconut Cream	28 grams/1oz	10	1	1
Olives	28 grams/1oz	4	0.5	1
Avocados	28 grams/1oz	4	2	1
Coconut Milk	28 grams/1oz	7	1	1

Almond Butter	28 grams/1oz	18	2	7
Brazil Nuts	28 grams/1oz	19	1	4
Heavy Cream, Full Fat	28 grams/1oz	10	1	1
Cheese, Cheddar	28 grams/1oz	9	1	7
Cheese, Blue	28 grams/1oz	8	1	6

What ought to be avoided are refined vegetable oils and trans fats, such as rapeseed oil, canola oil, margarine etc. They are more inflammatory and actually dangerous for our health. Also, the biggest reason why saturated fat is considered bad in the first place.

Top 5 recommendations for fat are:

- [MCT Oil](#)

- [Organic Extra Virgin Coconut Oil](#)

- [Extra Virgin Olive Oil](#)

- [Premium Avocado Oil](#)

- [Grass-Fed Butter](#)

Can you already feel yourself better? No more *fat free* yogurts, *zero fat* sauces, *reduced fat* meats that have lost all of their flavor or other nonsense. It's time to replace turkey bacon with real juicy pork bacon that triggers the *umami* taste of gods.

Getting into nutritional ketosis isn't easy. Initially, the body will reject this new fuel source and keeps on wanting to satisfy its glucose addiction. Sugar feeds parasites and promotes yeast infection in our gut. Having a big sweet tooth is the result of just that. The more we eat it the more we actually begin to crave because of certain dopamine receptors in our brain.

Simple carbohydrates make us want more of this stimulus by causing a rewarding feeling. Abstaining from sugar cleanses the body and liberates the mind from craving it. While in nutritional ketosis we're completely free from anything like that. The food we eat is already incredibly satisfying and we don't need anything sweetened.

Symptoms of Withdrawal

The biggest reason why the majority either fail or don't even start a ketogenic diet is that they are afraid of it.

After years of being fed a whole-grain diet and villainizing fat, they think that they're going to have a heart attack. Of course, if you were to eat randomly and not ditch the carbs, then you're going to have a bad time.

If they have decided to try it out, then they will also come across a lot of negative side effects. **The process of adaptation takes at least 2-3 weeks.** At first, you won't be able to experience almost any of the benefits, but will suffer from withdrawal symptoms.

This "keto flu" happens because the body doesn't know how to use fat for fuel. The brain will be screaming for energy and demands glucose. Eating carbs will put a cold halt to inducing ketosis and prevents any metabolic change.

This is where patience and perseverance come into play. The severity of it will depend on how addicted to sugar your body has been before. If you come from the background of the SAD diet, then it will take you longer than someone who is used to eating paleo and already used to less sugar.

During that period there will be some uncomfortable signs of withdrawal, such as dizziness, fatigue, slight headaches and the feeling of being hit with a club, which all pass away after a while.

Am I in Ketosis?

To know whether or not you're in ketosis you can measure your blood ketones using Ketostix. Optimal measurements are between 0,5 and 3,0 mMol. The same can be done with a glucometer. If you're fasting blood glucose is under 80 mg/dl and you're not feeling hypoglycemic then you're probably in ketosis. Ketoacidocis occurs over 10mMol, which is quite hard to reach.

What level of Ketosis is optimal?

Page 91: The Art and Science of Low Carbohydrate Performance
Jeff S. Volek and Stephen D. Phinney

BLOOD GLUCOSE CHART

Mg/DL	Fasting	After Eating	2-3 hours After Eating
Normal	80-100	170-200	120-140
Impaired Glucose	101-125	190-230	140-160
Diabetic	126+	220-300	200 plus

But there are a few problems with measuring ketones.

- Having elevated levels of ketones doesn't mean you're in ketosis.
- These urine strips are expensive and taking several measurements a day is very costly.

That's why we there's another way how to know you're in ketosis without strips. Elevated ketone levels don't necessarily mean ketosis. It might even be the opposite.

If we're not putting that fuel into use, then we're probably urinating it out. That's why urine strips are not ideal.

What we want to know as well is our blood sugar levels. Glucose and ketones are contradicting fuel sources. If one is elevated, then the other has to be decreased.

If we have high blood sugar levels, then we won't be able to use fat for fuel. We definitely won't be in ketosis.

There are a lot of additional symptoms of ketosis that occur during adaptation.

Water weight loss.

The biggest of which is probably fluid retention, or in this case, lack thereof. Carbohydrate molecules are very prone to binding together with liquids. Our body is made up of a lot of water and therefore can store a lot of it in our muscles.

Once you start restricting your carb intake, you'll lose a lot of water weight. It's not fat necessarily but just your excess sugar being flushed out.

You're thirsty.

What will follow is also increased thirst. This is caused by a loss in water weight to a certain extent. In addition to that, you'll want to drink more water because your body needs it.

The more water you drink, the less of it your body will store. While eating carbs, you're prone to depositing it because of increased liquid retention. Once you get flushed, you will be slightly dehydrated and have to compensate for it with increased water intake.

It's like you were dehydrated previously as well. Just that carbs prevented you from getting that thirsty.

Drink a lot of water. At least 8 cups a day. On a ketogenic diet or eating low carb, even more.

Keto breath.

The most infamous symptoms of ketosis is a smelly mouth. Once you're stored carbohydrates have been depleted you begin to use more fat for fuel.

During lipolysis (burning fatty acids in the Krebs cycle) we create a ketone body called acetone. Instead of using it for energy, we'll be excreting most of it in our urine and breath. That's how Ketostix work as well.

The smell is often described as "fruity", acidic or slightly rotten. If you've got an upcoming date, then be wary.

Metallic taste in your mouth

Because of the same reason we'll be having a slightly metallic or sweet taste in our mouth. It's acetone leaving its mark in our saliva and breath.

Stinky urine.

Acetone again being excreted by the body. The odor is quite strong. To be honest, it smells like acidic death. Your sweat can also have the same effects.

Because you'll be flushing out water, you'll experience urinating more often as well. Stay hydrated.

Slight headaches and fatigue.

During keto adaptation your body is going through a slight energy crisis. It still wants to use glucose but there's none around. It doesn't know how to burn fat for fuel yet and is therefore making you feel exhausted.

The initial period may cause headaches, sugar cravings, lethargy and muscle fatigue. Don't worry, these side effects will all pass away once you get fat adapted. This is also what makes people shy away from ketosis the most. They just don't have the patience.

Lack of appetite.

Next to all of these slightly uncomfortable symptoms, there are also amazing ones. The best of which is reduced appetite. You'll be eating a lot of fat, protein and fibrous vegetables, which are all the most satiating nutrients.

Because of that you'll almost never feel hungry and are constantly satisfied with your meals. You won't have to eat as often as well, because of your body burning fat for fuel.

After Adaptation

If you've eaten low carb for about 2-3 weeks, then you're probably in ketosis. At some point, you'll start to feel a lot better. In fact, better than ever before.

You'll experience.

- No hunger whatsoever.
- Mental clarity.
- High levels of energy at all times.
- Increased endurance.
- Reduced inflammation
- Reduced bloating.
- No sugar cravings.
- Improved sleep.
- Stable blood sugar levels.
- No muscle catabolism.
- Less fatigue during exercise, any other time as well, really.

This is what to expect once you've become fat adapted. You can use Ketostix to measure your progress. But it doesn't necessarily mean you're in ketosis *per se*. Follow your intuition first and foremost.

Do I Have to be in Ketosis?

Quantifying and measuring can turn into an obsession. Trust me, it's very frustrating to not see your blood glucose levels not being where you want them to be despite trying very hard. It can cause a lot of stress. At least that's how I felt during my initial adaptation period. That's why I wanted to show you how to get into ketosis without losing your mind.

To be honest, it doesn't matter whether or not you're in ketosis. It's not a magic pill that immediately turns you into a superhuman. Nor is it a badge of honor that you could wear. *"Oh, look at me, my blood ketone levels are in the optimal zone. Therefore, I'm better than you!"*

In my opinion we don't need nor should want to be in ketosis all of the time. It's a great tool to have in our metabolic arsenal but not the only one. I love eating keto because of how it makes me feel.

Unless you're diabetic or have any other medical condition, then you shouldn't worry about getting kicked out of ketosis.

Nutritional ketosis *per se* isn't the purpose of health and well-being. Being fat adapted and burning fat for fuel is a lot more important. This can be achieved by eating low carb as well. However, the initial period of keto adaptation is necessary for these pathways to be created.

Chapter IV
To Get Fat Adapted Don't Do This.

Going through the adaptation period is difficult but highly rewarding afterwards. Having done it quite a few times myself I can tell that it gets easier the more you do it. The more your body knows how to use fat for fuel the less side effects you'll have. My own experiments with ketosis have taught me a lot about nutrition and how to become more efficient with the fuel I'm using.

There are a lot of things that could potentially hinder adaptation, which I came to the conclusion of from my own experience. Before jumping in head first we need to keep in mind several important factors.

Too Many Carbs to Adapt

The biggest mistake we could make is to consume too many carbohydrates. They need to be restricted to less than 30 grams per day, without the fiber, for our body to enter ketosis.

The problem with most low carb diets is that they do not restrict their sugar intake enough for the body to completely convert over to fat burning. Even consuming slightly too much will keep us on the peripheral areas of keto adaptation. This is the worst place to be in because we will not be able to shift our metabolism into efficiently using ketones or get enough energy from glucose.

To get the most out of that amount we ought to be consuming only green leafy vegetables and not waste our allowance on things that don't satiate us as much.

Sugar hides itself in all shapes and form. Processed meat usually has added wheat or is cured in dextrose. Even though some foods might be keto friendly, such as heavy whipping cream, cheese and nuts, they still have a significant amount of sugar in them. That is why it's important to read the labels of everything that has one, as they can potentially spike our insulin. It almost resembles deciphering the complex linguistics of some ancient tablets.

How to Read Nutrition Labels

There are some national variations in terms of terminology, quantities and legislations but the core principles remain the same as long as we interpret the data according to our individual context. Put on your Indiana Jones' hat because this requires a lot of deciphering and linguistic work.

This is just a random example about what's most relevant and will guide you to making better decisions.

1. **The serving information.** We'll start from the very top. This will tell you the size of a single serving and the total amount of them per package. These are random

measurements not recommendations and the food companies can use them to trick uneducated readers.

2. **Calories per serving.** A bag of chips may have only 100 calories per serving, but the entire bag has 5 of them, totaling in 500 calories. I wouldn't bother making real interpretations based solely on this. The best way to understand this data is to adjust it to 100 grams instead.

3. **Macronutrient ratios.** Next check out all of the macros. It's important to also see what proportions each of them contain. Be aware of the amount of trans fats and sugars. In the case of carbohydrates note how much of it is fiber as it may differ from the actual soluble content. I would completely ignore the % of daily values because the public recommendations are not individualized and taken out of context. It's based on an average 2000 calorie diet and might be completely the opposite to what we need. We only want to know the amounts we will be consuming and adjust that according to our own demands.

4. **Micronutrients.** The same applies to the vitamins. There is not much use to knowing how many micronutrients we're getting. If anything, then they're more likely put there to distract the reader away from all of the other potential hazards and bring in more confusion. Our individual deficiencies play a role here as well and we don't necessarily need everything.

5. **Ingredients.** They have to be listed in order of quantity with the major ones coming first. Some of them should also have exact percentages and amounts. All of the allergens or hazards are bolded for faster recognition but it varies between countries. Make sure you read and understand all of them and steer away from the dangers.

In the United States if a food has less than 0,5 grams of trans fat in a serving, the label can have 0 grams of it. This hidden sources will add up if you eat too much and can be the hidden source of your problems. That's why it's important to also check the ingredient list for the actual contents for hydrogenated fats and vegetable oils.

Additionally, what needs to be counted towards the daily carbohydrate allowance is seasoning. Industrialized mixes like lemon pepper or table salt are already contaminated with dextrose and, therefore, ought to be avoided like wildfire.

Natural spices, like cinnamon, turmeric and ginger also have a minute carbohydrate content. We should be using them for their other medicinal benefits but be careful not to go overboard. This was one of the missing pieces of the puzzle that slowed down my adaptation the first time. I used to sprinkle seasoning on everything but didn't count them towards my daily carb allowance.

List of foods to avoid:

- All types of tubers, such as carrots, turnips, beetroot, potatoes.
- All grain products, such as rice, flour, wheat, barley, rye, quinoa.
- All legumes and lentils.
- All fruit, such as bananas, apples, oranges, grapes, watermelon etc.

- No yogurt with added sugar, no sodas, no milk, no chocolate, no cookies, no chips etc.

Too Much Protein, Bro

After eating too many carbohydrates, the next possible thing that hinders adaptation would be *glyconeogenesis*. Eating too much protein can convert even the juiciest of stakes into cake in our blood stream. What you don't need right away gets turned into sugar because during withdrawal every ounce of glucose is valuable. The body will sniff out whatever it can find.

However, for that to happen we would have to be consuming quite a lot. The recommended daily allowance for protein is already very low in comparison to what we would benefit from. How much we need depends on our weight and activity levels.

A sedentary person doesn't need nearly as much as someone who trains hard. If you're a small woman, then your requirements would be less than 100 grams per day. However, an athlete ought to be minimally consuming 0.8 grams per pound of lean body mass or 2 grams per kilogram, which is quite low and not nearly as much as the bodybuilding gurus tell us to eat.

The maximum we could get away with would be 1 g/pound. Anything higher than that will potentially turn into sugar. All kinds of whey powders and shakes are just another way to get money out of people by overemphasizing the importance of protein.

Ketosis is actually protein sparing because of the constant anabolic state we're in. Muscles will always have enough calories around and don't need to break down the body's own tissue and organs for energy.

After you've become fat adapted you don't have to worry about this as much. If you eat too much protein you'll get kicked out of ketosis, but only for a short period of time. Once a few hours have passed you'll re-enter the fat burning zone. However, eating excessive protein is bad for other aspects of your health, such as longevity and tumor growth. Better stick within the keto allowance.

__Not Enough Fat...What?__

Another mistake would be not eating enough fat. As weird as it might sound that could happen. By eliminating carbohydrates from the menu we need to have another fuel source to feed our hungry brain. This means putting butter and olive oil over everything. The lethargy and fatigue can be minimized by not adding caloric restriction on top of the adaptation process.

If we give our body more fat, it will inevitably have to accept it. Moreover, this will also promote the liver's production of additional ketone bodies. To be honest, there isn't a limit to how much fat we should consume. The more we do, the better for the induction of ketosis. What needs to be avoided, however, are the wrong types of fats, such as vegetable oils and trans fats, because of their inflammatory properties.

After all of the other macronutrients have been dialed in and potential infiltrations of sugar removed it's only a matter of time. It takes a lot of patience to get into ketosis. Quantifying with Ketostix or a glucometer would tell us about our progress but we shouldn't get caught up with the numbers. We can easily become consumed by it which would make things only worse.

Additional Factors

During the initial adaptation phase, we want to keep our stress levels as low as possible because it will stop us from adjusting to this massive change our body is going through. Quality nutrition, sleep, hydration, fresh air, exercise, being calm and centered are especially important at that time.

Drinking more than adequate amounts of water is very important. Carbs make the body hold onto liquids more easily because of their molecular structure. Once we deprive ourselves from glucose we will flush out a lot of water weight. This is perfectly normal but to prevent any negative consequences of that, we need to increase our hydration.

The recommendation is about 8 cups of water a day but it's not enough on keto. Drink at least 10 cups a day. At the same time, listen to your intuition and also look at the color of your urine.

If you're not thirsty, then don't feel obligated to drink more water.

URINE COLOR CHART

Hydrated

Dehydrated

Extremely Dehydrated
(consult a doctor)

Additionally, mineral intake with sodium is also vital. Electrolyte deficiencies will lead to muscle cramping, headaches and too much stress.

What's more, drinking too much water and peeing may make us excrete out our electrolytes more than we consume. That's why you should pay close attention to your urine color and how often you tend to go to the bathroom. If you do it every hour, then dial back on your water intake.

To make sure we keep things in check, we can drink water with a bit of good quality salt in it to improve our hydration and reduce cortisol levels, especially if we do it first thing in the morning.

One of the biggest things that gets neglected in our modern wired up lives is sleep. It's the time during which our body conducts all of its repair processes. Growth hormone is also released the most during the first few hours of shut-eye at about 11 PM.

Make sure you get about 7-8 hours of sleep a night because anything less will cause too much stress to the body. Inadequate amounts will lead to insulin resistance, too high blood glucose levels, fatigue, fat accumulation and muscle waste.

The best advice I can give you is to adjust your sleeping schedule to the circadian rhythm. This might not be possible but it's the ideal worth striving towards. The most optimal time to go to bed is at about 10PM. Waking up depends, but cortisol starts raising at about 5-7AM to wake us up naturally.

Noon 12:00
High alertness 10:00
Highest testosterone secretion 09:00
Bowel movement likely 08:30
Melatonin secretion stops 07:30
Sharpest rise in blood pressure 06:45
06:00
Lowest body temperature 04:30
02:00 Deepest sleep
00:00 Midnight
Best coordination 14:30
Fastest reaction time 15:30
Greatest cardiovascular efficiency and muscle strength 17:00
18:00
18:30 Highest blood pressure
19:00 Highest body temperature
21:00 Melatonin secretion starts
22:30 Bowel movements suppressed

To make sure you get a good night's sleep, you have to block out blue light exposure from your gadgets and technology. It will keep our subconscious mind up and suppresses melatonin, which is the sleep hormone. Start wearing blue light blocking glasses after 8PM and install a software called Flux on your computer.

First thing in the morning after waking up, you should drink at least 1 cup of water with about ½ teaspoons of either sea salt or rock salt in it. Make sure you mix it nicely with a spoon before because it will make the sodium crystals blend in with the liquid.

Therefore, we should maintain this zen-like attitude towards the whole experience and simply let things everything run their course. Rather than being frustrated or lethargic we have to accept it as it is. We can't control what happens to us but only our response to it.

It ought to be something we enjoy and can later reflect back upon as an opportunity to learn more about our own body. Don't stress out on your ketone levels either. There isn't a specific point where we will become fat adapted but eventually we'll simply get accustomed to this new alteration of our own biology.

Chapter V

Intermittent Fasting

A healthy lifestyle should also include some abstention from food. Fasting induces ketosis very rapidly within 2-3 days and is the most natural and quickest ways of doing it.

Ketone bodies may rise up to 70-fold during prolonged fasting[xxi]. Fasting also skyrockets human growth hormone exponentially within the first few days to maintain lean body mass and muscle tissue. Afterwards it does so less significantly because protein catabolism gets reduced to almost non-existent levels. In this state, the majority of the body's energy demands will be met by the use of free fatty acids and ketones.

Physiologically, fasting and ketosis are the 2 sides of the same coin. However, there are even more benefits that are characteristic specifically to fasting.

The benefits of intermittent fasting:

- Cellular repair and detoxification through a pathway called autophagy, which removes waste material from cells[xxii]
- Increased metabolism by 3.6-14% after 48 hours[xxiii]
- More insulin sensitivity[xxiv]
- Human growth hormone gets skyrocketed by 1300-2000%[xxv]
- Increased longevity and lifespan
- Cancer and tumor protection
- Bolstered brain power and protection against neurodegenerative disease

As you can see, most of the benefits, *sans autophagy,* can be achieved on a well-formulated ketogenic diet as well.

There are several ways we can structure our intermittent fasting.

Actually, it doesn't even matter when, as long as you simply do it. The length of the fast isn't as important either. After a certain amount of time we'll have reaped all of the benefits and can stop fasting, without going through several days.

Here are a few ways of doing it.

- **24-hour fast.** This is the most basic way. It doesn't even have to mean that you actually go through a day without eating. Simply have dinner in the evening, fast throughout the next day and eat dinner again. This one is also prescribed by the author of *Eat Stop Eat* Brad Pilon. The frequency depends on the person but once or twice a week should be the golden standard. An active person who trains hard should do it less often than a sedentary person.

- **16/8 time frame every day.** This is my favorite strategy, popularized by Martin Berkhan, which I'm doing daily. You fast for 16 hours and have a feeding window of 8. Simply skip breakfast and have it during lunch instead. By that time all of the HGH and other hormonal benefits will have reached their peak. It's also the time where our body has managed to digest and remove all of the food and waste from the previous day. In my opinion, we should all be following this. It's an optimal way of eating by consuming food only when it's necessary. We don't even have to be as strict with it. Instead of following 16/8 we can do 14/10, 18/6, 20/4 or whatever fits the situation. The point is to simply reduce the amount of time we spend in a fed state and to be fasting for the majority of the day.

- The Warrior Diet is a fasting protocol created by Ori Hofmekler. The entire concept is based around ancient warrior nations, such as the Spartans and Romans, who would be physically active throughout the day and only eat at night. At daylight they would only get a few bites here and there and would consume a lot of calories in the evening. This diet follows the 20/4 timeframe with one massive meal eaten at dinner.

- **Fasting for several days.** Although very effective for weight loss, I don't see immense benefits in doing this for healthy individuals. Autophagy and detoxification will certainly increase but I would like to think that similar results will be achieved with daily intermittent fasting, such as the 16/8 window. The frequency might actually be a lot better than the intensity. However, doing a fast for several days at least once a year sounds like a wise idea, as it will completely detoxify the body and will also clear metal toxicity.

- **Breakfast and dinner.** As a final resort you can follow the pattern of 50-50, meaning you have breakfast early in the morning, go through the day without eating and have dinner. This way you'll fast for about 8-10 hours and actually do it twice in one 24-hour period. It's not ideal but still better than 6 meals a day. At least you'll be able to not become too dependent of the food and can get the most of the benefits.

There are also approaches like *The 5:2 Diet* and *Alternate Day Fasting*, which include fasting but allow the consumption of about 500 calories on days of abstention. I wouldn't recommend this, because caloric restriction won't allow all of the physiological benefits of fasting to kick in. You want to shock the body and go straight to zero for the greatest effects.

Based on my research and experimentation, the most effective way to do this is through *Intermittent Fasting and Feasting*, which is also the title of one the books I've written about the topic. In its core, it resembles a lot the Warrior Diet, but is slightly different. It's actually better, because it incorporates periods of undereating and overfeeding with nutritional ketosis.

Basically, you skip breakfast, fast for about 15-17 hours until noon and have a very small ketogenic meal of about 300-500 calories. As a result, the insignificant impact on blood sugar levels will prolong your fasting period even further and makes you more ketogenic. After that, you wait about 5-6 hours and have a big dinner. You'll still be eating keto foods but in larger quantities.

The advantage to this is 3-fold.

- By skipping breakfast, you allow your body to conduct detoxifying and autophagy.

- At noon, your HGH production will have increased and having a small meal will give you more energy to.

- Keeping yourself slightly underfed throughout the day sends a signal to the body to speed up nutrient partitioning and protein synthesis. By overfeeding at dinner you'll utilize your food more efficiently and supercompensate for the abstinence.

Another thing to consider is protein fasting. In a nutshell, you occasionally reduce your daily protein intake dramatically, almost to a zero. It's a great tool to reduce inflammation, kick-start weight loss and to protect yourself against tumors, cancer and aging.

By doing protein fasting once a week, you're allowing your body to induce *autophagy*. You'll be self-digesting your own tissue. It might seem like you're cannibalizing yourself and starving, but in reality *autophagy* is required to maintain lean body mass and it actually inhibits the breakdown of muscle in adults[xxvi].

It also improves mitochondrial functioning, resulting in better sleep. *Autophagy* is required for healthy brain cell mitochondria[xxvii]. Regular fasting does the trick as well, but regularly limiting your protein intake is another great way to do this. This makes your cells find every possible way to recycle proteins endogenously. At the same time, they bind and excrete toxins that are hidden in your cell's cytoplasm[xxviii].

Being chronically protein deficient is horrible for the brain and body. The trick is to do it intermittently, like with fasting. After skipping protein intake completely (24-hour fast) or reducing your intake close to zero (about 15 grams), you'll supercompensate for that scarcity and increase its utilization.

Doing some form of intermittent fasting daily in concert with keto is one of the greatest health hacks there is. It doesn't even feel like an abstention if we structure it strategically. That's why the minimum fasting window I would recommend for everyone is 14-16 hours.

Here's how to maximize your daily intermittent fasting and ketogenic eating.

- Instead of having breakfast first thing in the morning, continue to fast for a few hours.

- Drink a lot of water to keep yourself hydrated. Either add some salt or drink mineral water.

- Wait until you get hungry and then drink either black coffee or tea.

- Fast for about 14-18 hours until noon. HGH and other hormones will have peaked by that time.

- Before you eat, have a glass of warm lemon water. The citric acid will promote the creation of good digestive enzymes and prepares your gut for digestion.

- Break your fast with something small. Eating a big meal will put too much stress on your intestines. Have a few eggs and vegetables with some fat. You shouldn't feel the need to eat more than 300-500 calories

- Wait a few hours and continue eating the rest of your calories.

To be honest, the majority of the benefits will be covered with that short time period. However, having a 24-hour fast once a week and a 48-hour one every few months will do your health an extraordinary service.

Chapter VI
A Definitive Guide to
Starting the Ketogenic Diet

Now that we've covered all we need to know about nutritional ketosis, it's prime time to actually implement it.

We've covered all of the basics we need to know about nutrition and ketosis. With the information you've received, you're already more knowledgeable than the majority of people. It's an essential and vital skill to know what effect food has on us and how to optimize it.

What we eat has a lot more profound impact on us than we think. High end performance and a good quality life require us to take care of our body.

It starts with the gut. Our stomach is the closest point of contact we have with the world and is the most sensitive to external stimulus. What we put into our mouth will travel down our throat into the intestines where it will be used appropriately. If what you swallowed was food, hopefully, your body will release hydrochloric acid (HCA), which begins the digestion process.

Gut integrity and health is associated the most with bodily inflammation levels, which is the greatest predictor of overall health and longevity. Inhabited by millions of bacteria, our microbiome operates like a second brain that is constantly communicating with the rest of the body and sending out signals about what processes to conduct at any given moment.

Gut Flora
- Key role in nutrition
- Produces digestive enzymes
- Synthesize vitamins

Immune System
- Starts in the mouth, all the way to the intestines
- **90% is in the gut**

By being inflamed we will begin to suffer joint pain, brain fog and overall slothfulness. The 90% of our body's population is non-human and they control our appetite, hormones, metabolism and mood. It is essential to keep our gut clean and happy so that we too could feel great.

The reason why this is so important is that it will determine how well you're going to do on this ketogenic diet. If you neglect your gut, your brain and overall life will suffer.

It Starts with a Healthy Gut

Dark leafy greens are excellent sources of fiber, vitamins, enzymes and minerals that feed the good gut microbiome. Adding in excellent sources of fat and protein we are allowing our food to be digested properly and do it with ease without causing inflammation.

On the other hand, if we were to consume refined carbohydrates or whole grains then we will eventually get leaky gut, which is a syndrome where the phytates and gluten compounds destroy the intestinal walls, allowing the waste to flood our blood stream. As a result, we will suffer all of the diseases we are trying to avoid. Gluten-free might be considered a fad by some, but it's based on real science and physiology.

One thing to avoid entirely is the use of antibiotics. If you're taking some, then I advise you to find a better solution because these drugs kill all bacteria, the good and the bad. Also, you will cause gut irritation and excessive stress. Your body will heal itself from almost anything over time. Mostly our own behavior puts a halt to it. What we can do is assist the process.

Start eating an anti-inflammatory ketogenic diet. By removing processed food from your menu and eating plenty of healthy vegetables, fat and meat, you're already solving the issue to a great degree.

In addition to that, eating fermented foods is a must. You should eat at least some form of it every day. As weird as it might sound, your plate has to be full of nutrition as well as crawling with bacteria. The best sources are sauerkraut, pickles, kimchi, tempeh, Kombucha, raw milk, raw yogurt and kefir. You can make all of them at home yourself. Commercial products aren't nearly as effective and can have added sugar in them.

Here's how to make your own sauerkraut.

Ingredients

- Cabbage

- An empty jar

- Salt, pepper, or any other spices you like.

- A food processor.

Preparation

- Use the food processor to shred the cabbage.

- Pack it tightly together with the spices into the jar.

- The released liquid creates its own brining solution.

- Leave the jar open and put a rock or something heavy on top of the cabbage for extra pressure.

- Keep it at room temperature at somewhere with access to air.

- After a few days, the cabbage will have fermented and is ready to be eaten.

What Changes You Should Make

Start taking care of your gut, eat fermented foods and pay more attention to your overall inflammation levels. If you feel worse after eating something, then you probably shouldn't eat it again.

The ketogenic diet works so great because you'll be cleaning your body and resetting it back to its primal functioning. You'll learn more about how you react to different nutrients and how to optimize your intake accordingly. It's not worth it to feel anything less than great.

Here are some additional changes we need to make to start a ketogenic lifestyle.

- **Swap out your pantry.** Get rid of all of your whole grain breads, pastas, cereal, oatmeal, potatoes, fruit, sugar, rice etc. You don't need to have them in your house if you're not going to eat them. At least lose them for the time being. They can only hinder your process. If there are only keto foods around, then you won't even get the thought of wanting to eat carbohydrates. You begin to crave carbs only after you take a bite of them. Pre-empt that in advance like a strategic genius.

- **Buy a lot of healthy ketogenic food.** To replace the carbs, go to a supermarket and stack up on some staple nutrients that you'll be consuming from now on. It might seem like keto is overly restrictive but in reality there is quite a lot of variation in the diet. Some of the essential ingredients you should stock up on are.

    o Extra Virgin Olive Oil– Make sure you get it in a dark bottle. You don't want to expose it to sunlight or heat, as it will go rancid and cause oxidative damage. Don't use it on a frying pan either. Use it only as cold dressing.

o <u>Extra Virgin Coconut Oil</u> – The best fat for cooking is coconut oil because its smoking point is 350°F/175°C. It's also full of medium-chain triglycerides, which are fatty acid chains with medium length bonds and can be quickly converted to energy.

o **Frozen vegetables.** To get the most nutrients from your food, you should always try to eat it as fresh as possible. Moments after picking up a vegetable, the micronutrient content begins to diminish. However, refrigerating food will maintain its freshness, as it gets flash frozen right on the field. Buy a lot of frozen broccoli, cauliflower, kale, Brussels sprouts, green beans etc.

o **Frozen meat.** The same applies to animal products. You don't want to eat something that has gone rancid or has stayed on the shelf for too long. Exceeding the expiration date won't do you no harm, as the bacteria count will actually increase. However, you should still stock up on some frozen meat. Buy frozen pork chops, chicken thighs, organ meats, fish and beef.

- **Stack up on healthy seasoning.**

  o <u>Pink Himalayan Rock Salt</u> – Hydration and electrolyte balance are incredibly important on a ketogenic diet. By ditching carbs, your body will flush out a lot of liquids, which needs to be compensated by drinking more water and increasing your sodium intake. Ordinary table salt is contaminated with unhealthy nitrates. A good quality sea or pink salt also has a higher magnesium content, which is an essential nutrient to have.

  o **Turmeric.** One of the best spices we can use is curcumin or turmeric. It has a lot of medicinal properties, such as anti-inflammatory compounds, increase of antioxidants and brain health. Also, it fights and prevents many diseases, such as Arthritis,

Alzheimer's and even cancer. In addition to that, it tastes amazing and can be added to everything. I sprinkle it on all foods and run out quite quickly which is why I also buy it in bulk so that it's cheaper. You can also take a capsule.

- **Ginger.** Continuing on with turmeric's brother. It has almost as much health benefits. In addition to that, it lowers blood sugar levels, fights heart disease, treats chronic indigestion, may reduce menstrual pain for women, lowers cholesterol and heals muscle pain. Once again, bulk or capsule.

- **Cinnamon.** These three create the most important natural spices we should be eating on a daily basis. They're incredibly cheap and easy to come by yet have amazing health as well as performance enhancing benefits. Moreover, they all make food taste amazing. Cinnamon falls into the same category as ginger and turmeric - superfoods, because it truly empowers us. In addition to the same medicinal properties it also increases insulin sensitivity, fights neurodegenerative disease and bacterial infections. What's best about it is that it can be added to not only salty foods but on desserts as well. I even add it to my coffee. The best to use is Ceylon or „true" cinnamon.

- **Calculate your macros.** You don't need to take this to neurotic levels. However, during the initial few weeks of adaptation, you should pay some attention to this. Weigh your food for a few days and follow the ketogenic macronutrient ratios.

    o **Carbs.** The total caloric proportion should be about 5-10% NET, which doesn't include the fiber. This will fall somewhere between 30-50 grams per day. Carb tolerances vary between individuals and you should know where yours lies. The lower your carb intake the faster will ketosis be induced. After the adaptation period you can get away with eating slightly more and don't have to worry about it that much.

- **Protein.** The ketogenic diet is moderate in protein with 15-25% of total calories. If you're a sedentary person, then your demands will be even less. As a general guideline stick to somewhere between 0.7 to 1.3 grams per pound of lean body mass. If you're a hard-charging athlete, your needs will be higher.

- **Fat.** The rest of your calories will come from fat, more than 70-80%. Eating more will not hurt your keto-adaptation. However, it's still a source of dense calories. If you're trying to lose weight, then you can't do so by eating at a surplus. You still have to be at a negative energy balance. The reason why keto works so great for this is that the satiety factor will by default make you eat less.

You can also use this free online macro calculator http://keto-calculator.ankerl.com/

Keto Shopping List

You're going to have to swap out all of your pantry. Here are the keto-safe groceries for all macronutrients, including their actual caloric content.

Food Source	Calories	Fats (g)	Net Carbs (g)	Protein (g)
Protein				
Bacon, 1 slice (~ 8g), baked	44	3.5	0	2.9
Beef, Sirloin Steak, 1 ounce, broiled	69	4	0	7.7

Beef, Ground, 5% fat, 1 ounce, broiled	44	1.7	0	6.7
Beef, Ground, 15% fat, 1 ounce, broiled	70	4.3	0	7.2
Beef, Ground, 30% fat, 1 ounce, broiled	77	5.1	0	7.1
Beef, Bottom Round, 1 ounce, roasted	56	2.7	0	7.6
Chicken, white meat, 1 ounce	49	1.3	0	8.8

Chicken, dark meat, 1 ounce	58	2.8	0	7.8
Egg, 1 large, 50 g	72	4.8	0.4	6.3
Fish, Raw, Cod, 1 ounce	20	0.1	0	4.3
Fish, Raw, Flounder, 1 ounce	20	0.6	0	3.5
Fish, Raw, Sole, 1 ounce	20	0.6	0	3.5
Fish, Raw, Salmon, 1 ounce	40	1.8	0	5.6
Ham, smoked, 1 ounce	50	2.6	0	6.4

Hot dog, beef, 1 ounce	92	8.5	0.5	3.1
Lamb, ground, 1 ounce, broiled	80	5.6	0	7
Lamb chop, boneless, 1 ounce, broiled	67	3.9	0	7.3
Pork chop, bone-in, 1 ounce, broiled	65	4.1	0	6.7
Pork ribs, ribs, 1 ounce, roasted	102	8.3	0	6.2
Scallops, 1 ounce, steamed	31	0.2	1.5	5.8

Shrimp, 1 ounce, cooked	28	0.1	0	6.8
Tuna, 1 ounce, cooked	52	1.8	0	8.5
Turkey Breast, 1 ounce, roasted	39	0.6	0	8.4
Veal, roasted, 1 ounce	42	1	0	8
Vegetables				
Asparagus, cooked, 1 ounce	6	0.1	0.6	0.7
Avocado, 1 ounce	47	4.4	0.6	0.6

Broccoli, chopped, cooked, 1 ounce	10	0.1	1.1	0.7
Carrots, baby, 1 ounce, raw	10	0	1.5	0.01
Cauliflower, chopped, cooked, 1 ounce	7	0.1	0.5	0.5
Celery, 1 ounce, raw	5	0	0.3	0.7
Cucumber, 1 ounce, raw	4	0	1	0.2
Garlic, 1 clove (3 grams)	4	0	1	0.2

Green beans, cooked, 1 ounce	10	0.1	1.3	0.5
Mushrooms, button, 1 ounce, raw	6	0.2	0.6	0.9
Onion, green, 1 ounce, chopped, raw	9	0	1.3	0.5
Onion, white, 1 ounce, chopped, raw	11	0	2.1	0.3
Bell Pepper, Green, 1 ounce, raw	6	0	0.8	0.2
Pickles, dill, 1 ounce	3	0	0.4	0.2

Romaine lettuce, 1 ounce	5	0.1	0.3	0.4
Butterhead lettuce, 1 ounce	4	0.06	0.3	0.4
Shallots, raw, 1 ounce	20	0	3.9	0.7
Snow peas, 1 ounce, cooked	24	0	2.8	1.5
Spinach, 1 ounce, raw	7	0.1	0.4	0.8
Squash, Acorn, baked, 1 ounce	16	0	2.9	0.3
Squash, Butternut, baked, 1 ounce	11	0	2.1	0.3

Squash, Spaghetti, 1 ounce, cooked	8	0.1	1.4	0.2
Tomato, raw, 1 ounce	5	0	0.8	0.3
Dairy				
Buttermilk, whole, 1 ounce	18	0.9	1.4	0.9
Cheese, Blue, 1 ounce	100	8.2	0.7	6.1
Cheese, Brie, 1 ounce	95	7.9	0.1	5.9
Cheese, Cheddar, 1 ounce	114	9.4	0.4	7.1

Cheese, Colby, 1 ounce	110	9	0.7	6.7
Cheese, Cottage, 2%, 1 ounce	24	0.7	1	3.3
Cheese, Cream, block, 1 ounce	97	9.7	1.1	1.7
Cheese, Feta, 1 ounce	75	6	1.2	4
Cheese, Monterey Jack, 1 ounce	106	8.6	0.2	7
Cheese, Mozzarella, whole milk, 1 oz	85	6.3	0.6	6.3

Cheese, Parmesan, hard, 1 ounce	111	7.3	0.9	10.1
Cheese, Swiss, 1 ounce	108	7.9	1.5	7.6
Cheese, Marscapone, 1 ounce	130	13	1	1
Cream, half-n-half, 1 ounce	39	3.5	1.3	0.9
Cream, heavy, 1 ounce	103	11	0.8	0.6
Cream, Sour, full fat, 1 ounce	55	5.6	0.8	0.6

Milk, whole, 1 ounce	19	1	1.5	1
Milk, 2%, 1 ounce	15	0.6	1.5	1
Milk, skim, 1 ounce	10	0	1.5	1
Nuts and seeds				
Almonds, raw, 1 ounce	170	15	3	6
Brazil Nuts, raw, 1 ounce	186	19	1	4
Cashews, raw, 1 ounce	160	13	7	5
Chestnuts, raw, 1 ounce	55	0	13	0

Chia Seeds, raw, 1 ounce	131	10	0	7
Coconut, dried, unsweetened, 1 ounce	65	6	2	1
Flax Seeds, raw, 1 ounce	131	10	0	7
Hazelnuts, raw, 1 ounce	176	17	2	4
Madadamia Nuts, raw, 1 ounce	203	21	2	2
Peanuts, raw, 1 ounce	157	13	3	7
Pecans, raw, 1 ounce	190	20	1	3

Pine Nuts, raw, 1 ounce	189	20	3	4
Pistachios, raw, 1 ounce	158	13	5	6
Pumpkin Seeds, raw, 1 ounce	159	14	1	8
Sesame Seeds, raw, 1 ounce	160	14	4	5
Sunflower Seeds, raw, 1 ounce	150	11	4	3
Walnuts, raw, 1 ounce	185	18	2	4

Superfoods

On the other hand, there are also some additional "superfoods" we can consume. They are slightly less conventional and harder to find. Nevertheless, they are incredibly empowering and take it to the next level. Occasionally using them will yield great results.

First off, it's important to understand what we mean by "superfoods." Broccoli and turmeric fight cancer and reduce inflammation, eggs and salmon have omega-3s and DHA and can be considered as such. Because of the benefits we get from them, they are already a part of the list. However, they lack that one last push that would twist the entire thing over the top.

A superfood for a superhuman would have to be something that transcends their health and performance past our normal capacities and reach levels of post-optimal wellbeing.

Here's a list of some TRUE superfoods.

- **Blueberries.** Why? They're full of phytonutrients, that neutralize free radicals (agents that cause aging and cell damage). High antioxidant content also protects against cancer and reduces the effects of Alzheimer's and Parkinson's disease. They're brain food that improves cognitive functioning and memory. At the same time, it reduces the risk of heart disease and muscle damage from exercise.

- **Cacao.** Not hot chocolate, but raw cacao nibs. They can improve your memory, reduce heart disease, increase fat oxidation, boost immunity and grant a lot of energy. The Incas considered it the drink of the gods. Raw cacao contains 20 times more antioxidants than blueberries and 119 times more than bananas. Processed chocolate is made with roasted cocoa, milk, sugar and trans fats that block the absorption of antioxidants. Organic more than 80% dark chocolate can have the same benefits as raw cacao.

- Chia seeds. A very popular superfood because of its nutrient density and easy digestion. Aztec warriors ate chia seeds before battle for high energy and endurance. A spoonful was said to sustain them for 24 hours. In the Mayan language, "Chia" means "strength." These seeds are rich in fiber, omega-3s, protein, vitamins and minerals, such as copper, zinc and potassium. They will boost our metabolism, protect against heart disease, build muscle and increase fat burning. To get the most nutrition out of them you have to soak them in water for a few hours before consumption.

- **Algae.** It's a complex superfood that can be found in green, blue-green or brown seaweed. The health benefits are quite amazing: stronger immune system, increased white blood cell count and better gut flora. Blue-green algae like Chlorella or Spirulina is a source of vitamin B12 and 22 other amino acids. Brown algae contains Fuxoaxanthin that promotes fat burning.

- Bee pollen. Made by honeybees, it is one of the most nourishing foods Mother Nature can provide us with, as it contains almost all of the essential nutrients needed by humans. It's rich in amino acids, vitamins, including B-complex, and folic acid. Bee pollen is richer in protein than any animal source and half of it is directly used by the body. One teaspoon consists of over 2,5 billion (that's 9 zeros) flower pollen grains. Talk about micronutrient density. The benefits include: enhanced energy, smoother skin, high amounts of antioxidants, allergy reduction, improved digestion, stronger immune and cardiovascular system.

Start implementing these strategies here and you'll be living the ketogenic lifestyle. Buy good quality food, take care of your gut, change some of your eating habits and do intermittent fasting. You'll be off to achieving optimal health and wellbeing.

Chapter VII

The Ketogenic Cookbook

With the information in previous chapters we can immediately start eating delicious low carb meals that will eventually make us fat adapted. I've outlined the list of foods for you but you may still have some questions.

To give you an idea about what to cook during the adaptation phase and later, I'm going to give you a few recipes to get you started. The best thing about it is that you don't have to even give up some of your favourite high carb foods and can easily replace some of the ingredients with keto friendly substitutes.

The Ultimate Breakfast

The most classical and satiating meal we could have are eggs and bacon. They have a lot of fat and protein with the right nutritional profile for high end performance. Additionally, we want some fiber and more fat. Even though I would recommend eating eggs for DHA and cholesterol it might not be possible because of allergies. The substitute for that would be oily fish such as sardines, salmon, trout etc. The omega-3 fatty acids and EPA are even more beneficial for our cognition.

- **Ingredients:**
    - 3 Eggs
    - 1 slice of bacon or 1 oz/28g of fish/sausage
    - 1oz/28g of spinach/collard greens/broccoli/cabbage
    - 1 tbsp butter/lard/ghee/coconut oil
    - Optional additives would be cheese or avocado.
    - The spices would be pink Himalayan salt or regular sea salt, black pepper, turmeric, ginger, Cayenne pepper, cinnamon.
- **Preparation:** Either fry your eggs in a lot of butter, poach or boil them. Don't use too much heat as it will damage the nutrients. Throw in the bacon and mix the spinach in the same grease to coat it with fat.

Approximate calories: 450-500 calories (35g protein/40g fat/2g carbs)

To wash it all down with we would also want something to drink. I'm going to share with you my secret recipe that will change your life forever.

Fatty Egg Yolk Coffee

The name of this recipe might be somewhat shocking. Don't worry, you'll change your opinion once you've tasted it. It's not entirely my own idea and I must say kudos to Dave Asprey the Bulletproof executive. However, my own version of it is even better. If you don't drink coffee you can also use tea as a substitute.

- **Ingredients:**

    - Coffee/tea

    - 1 tbsp of butter/coconut oil/heavy cream/MCT oil

    - 1 whole egg

    - 1 tsp of raw cacao nibs, coconut flakes, Chaga mushroom, kelp powder and Chia seeds

    - 1/4 of an avocado seed, chopped. Yes, the avocado seed is very nutritious. You won't even notice the taste and will love the crunch it brings to your drink.

    - 1 tsp of cinnamon, turmeric, black pepper, sea salt and ginger

- **Preparation:**

    - Brew your beverage and let it simmer for a while.

    - Put the egg in your cup and break it down. If it stays in tact it will poach once you add the hot water.

    - Throw in some cacao nibs, coconut flakes, chia seeds, about 5-10 grams each.

- Chaga mushroom and sea kelp powder, 1/2 teaspoon each because they're quite intense in flavor.

- Add 1 teaspoon of butter, coconut oil, heavy cream or MCT oil – which one you like most.

- Chop down the avocado seed into tiny parts with a knife and put them in the cup.

- Sprinkle in cinnamon, turmeric, ginger, black pepper and sea salt. You can also try out Cayenne pepper for an extra kick.

- Then mix it vigorously with a spoon or use a blender to create a nice froth on the surface. Using a blender will break the avocado seeds and other ingredients into an amazing mixture. Shaken not stirred, please.

- Take a sip and be amazed.

Approximate calories: 250 (10g protein/20g fat/2g carbs)

It looks very appealing and has some pools of grease on the surface. Taste it and be amazed as all of your taste buds will fire up. This beverage gives instant and long lasting energy for hours. You won't experience any crash that accompanies drinking coffee either because the fat slows down the release of caffeine. There won't be any quick spike or drop and the brain will function at its best. All of the neurons will light up with joy and be satisfied.

Bone Broth Soup

One of the biggest downsides to eating keto is that some mineral deficiencies might occur. That isn't caused by the lack of variety in the diet but by the low nutritional quality of our soils and vegetables. To circumvent that we would have to take some supplements.

However, there is another way. It's even better and a great way to get in touch with our primal side. When a hunter-gatherer caught an animal nothing was wasted. Meat was a precious source of calories and they ate everything that was edible. Instead of trimming off the fat they went for the good stuff. Liver, kidneys, heart, bone marrow, skin with fat on – those are the most nutritious parts. It's only in today's contemporary society where people get disgusted by them. Culture depicts organ meat as putrid and the lean bits as something pure whereas we would be better off by neglecting none. This recipe transcends this dichotomy between the wild and domesticated by incorporating an ancestral practice into our menu.

- **Ingredients:**
    - Bones of a grass-fed and organically raised animal (chicken drumsticks, beef collar, wild boar bones etc.). Healthy animals will have stronger skeletomuscular structure.
    - Onions, garlic.
    - Optionally some organ meats such as: heart, kidneys, liver, chicken gizzards etc.
    - Spices: laurel-leafs, unground pepper and coarse sea salt.
- **Preparation:**

- Grab a big pot of water and throw in the ingredients. In order to get all of the minerals from the bones they need to be boiled for several hours on low heat. The longer they do the better. Put it on the stove at the beginning of the day and just let it sit there.
- Add the organ meats only during the last hour of preparation as they would simply turn to pudding.
- After a while the bones will begin to break down. Joints and tendons are the best because they have a lot of connective tissue attached to them. That's what we're after – the ligaments and the marrow inside. Once that happens the water will turn into a pool of fat and grease which tastes amazing.
- Drops of liquid begin to float the surface and give the soup its flavor. It can be used as a basis for other types of cooking or simply drank as a beverage.
- Storing it is easy as it will turn gelatinous after cooling down which can then be re-heated afterwards.

Approximate calories per 1 cup of soup: 110(5g protein/10g fat/0g carbs).

The bone broth soup is a great way to get in all of the essential minerals and nutrients we need from animals. Not only is it tasty and heart-warming but also very good for the gut. It reduces overall inflammation and promotes the strength of our joints because of the marrow.

Meaty Vegetable Roast-Feast

This is one of the best staple dinners we could ever have. It's quick and super easy to make with little to no effort involved.

The actual ingredients aren't as important as we can use anything. What matters are only the amounts and the idea.

- **Ingredients:**
    - Some source of fatty meat. Beef, pork chops, chicken wings, thighs etc.
    - Some source of leafy green vegetables. Cabbage, cauliflower, spinach, broccoli, collard greens etc.
    - Some source of extra fat. Butter, lard, ghee, olive oil etc.
    - Spices according to your liking.
- **Preparation:**
    - Grab a pan and add all of the ingredients by placing the greens on the bottom and the meat on top. Sprinkle bits of coarse sea salt on the meat so it would melt into it. Additionally, you can squeeze some lemon juice as well. Pour a bit of water into the bottom. Don't add any extra fat yet.
    - Put it all in the oven and let it cook for about 30-45 minutes. As its starting to be finished throw some butter on top. Don't heat olive oil because it will

oxidize and cause inflammation. Use it afterwards as dressing instead.

- o Mix all of the vegetables inside the fat. As a sider you can add some avocados or nuts. Dinner is served.

Approximate calories for 1 pound of dish: 750(50g protein/60g fat/6g carbs).

Kale Chips

Despite the low variety of foods on keto we can still use our creativity and come up with new ways to substitute the things we love. We can easily make crunchy chips using healthy ingredients that taste equally as good.

- **Ingredients:**
    - Some sort of leafy fibrous greens. Kale, savoy cabbage, bok choy, collard greens etc.
    - Seasoning according to preference.
    - 2 tbsp of olive oil
- **Preparation:**
    - Wash the vegetables and cut the leaves into smaller pieces.
    - Distribute them evenly on a pan and add seasoning.
    - Don't add too much water into the bottom as it will make the greens too soft.
    - Put the pan in the oven and bake for about 30-45 minutes on high heat.
    - It's finished when the leaves will turn brown and crunchy.
    - 10 minutes before taking them out, drizzle them with olive oil.

Approximate calories for 100g of chips: 100 calories (5g protein/7g fat/1g carbs).

Cauliflower Pizza

The most amazing and versatile food at our disposal on keto is cauliflower. It can be used to substitute almost anything we're used to having: mashed potatoes, rice and pizza. This recipe will teach you how to have your gluten-free-low-carb crust that fits ketosis perfectly.

- **Ingredients:**
    - 1 head of Cauliflower

- 2-3 Eggs
- 1 cup of Tomatoes
- ½ cup of Cheese
- 1 oz/25g of olives
- Seasoning and herbs of your choosing.

- **Preparation:**
  - Take the entire head of a cauliflower and cut off the florets.
  - In a food processor shred them all into bits and pieces.
  - Add in an egg or two and blend the mixture.
  - Spread the mixture on a pan and put it in the oven for 30 minutes at 375 F/190 C.
  - This will turn into a crust and creates texture.
  - Add the tomatoes and cheese on top and let it cook for a while until ready.

The same can be done with zucchini as well. Instead of it being pizza they look like boats instead. Simply cut the vegetable in half and add the other ingredients. Cook it in the oven until the cheese starts to melt down and you'll have a quick meal.

Approximate calories for the entire pizza: 900 (50g protein/40g fat/20g carbs).

Approximate calories for ¼ of the pizza: 250 (15g protein/10g fat/5g carbs).

Cheesy Tomato Soup

We don't have to drink bone broth by itself but can use it as a basis for other dishes as well. This recipe is perfect for that and tastes amazing. It will heal our gut and bring warmth into our heart.

- **Ingredients:**
    - Chicken bone broth with 2 drumsticks.
    - ½ cups of Cauliflower or broccoli.
    - 2 cups of Tomatoes.
    - 2 tablespoons of Soft cheese.
    - Optional: ¼ cups of coconut milk or heavy cream.
    - Basil leaves.
    - Seasoning according to liking.
- **Preparation:**
    - Put the drumsticks in the hot water and let it simmer for a while. The meat will cook quite easily and the

tendons break down faster because of their low density.

- o Chop down the tomatoes and let them be squashed.

- o Steam the vegetables until soft and smash them.

- o Add the seasoning and cheese to the vegetable blend.

- o Pour in coconut milk or heavy cream to make it thicker and consistent.

- o Stir it all up on a saucepan and let the cheese melt down.

- o Pour together the broth with the mixture and tomatoes.

- o Add the extra basil leaves and *voila!*

Approximate calories: 450(25g protein/30g fat/10g carbs).

Bacon and Egg Muffins

If you like to eat breakfast then I'm not going to stop you from doing so. Whatever suits your condition. Maybe you like to cook in the morning and do nothing else. In that case, the following recipes are for the more serious keto chef.

- **Ingredients**
    - 2 tbsp of heavy cream
    - 5oz/120g mushrooms, chopped

- 2 medium tomatoes, chopped
- 6 slices of bacon
- 4 eggs
- ¼ cup cheddar cheese, grated
- Seasoning according to preference

- **Preparation**
    - Preheat the oven to 375 degrees F (190 degrees C).
    - Cook the bacon strips on a frying pan on medium to low heat until crisp.
    - Use the bacon fat to grease the muffin cups.
    - Place one slice of bacon into each muffin cup so that the bacon lines the edges of the cup, like in a circle.
    - Beat the eggs and cream together, then pour them into muffin cups.
    - Bake in the oven until the muffins get slightly moist on top, which takes about 20 minutes. Season them with salt and pepper. Cover them with grated cheese and continue baking for about 5 minutes until melted.
    - Let the muffins cool down a bit and then remove them from the cups.

- Enjoy small mouth-sized bites!

Approximate calories: 1000-1200 (90g protein/100g fat/2g carbs)

Approximate calories per muffin: 220 (15g protein/17g fat/0.5g carbs).

This recipe covered 6 muffins but you can change the quantities as much as you'd like. It's simple – 1 bacon strip for each cup.

Coconut Cream Porridge

It's thought that oatmeal is incredibly healthy. Well, it might be, but it's definitely not optimal because of gluten and the phytates found in whole grains.

Nevertheless, there's still a way to have a bowl of keto porridge that tastes equally as good and doesn't come with any negative effects.

- **Ingredients**
    - 1 cup of coconut cream
    - 1 oz of almonds (about 20), ground or whole
    - 1 teaspoon of cinnamon and Stevia (optional)
    - 1 teaspoon of coconut flakes
    - A pinch of nutmeg
- **Preparation**
    - Heat the coconut cream on a saucepan on medium until it forms a liquid.
    - Add the almonds, coconut flakes and stevia
    - Mix well and keep stirring for a few minutes until it begins to thicken.

- o Add the cinnamon, nutmeg and taste.
- o Serve hot.

Approximate calories: 750 calories (15g protein/70g fat/15g carbs)

Bacon Brussel Sprouts

Another bacon recipe. It's just so delicious.

- **Ingredients**
    - o 3 slices bacon
    - o 3 cups of Brussels sprouts cut in half
    - o 1 tablespoon of garlic powder
    - o Sea salt

- **Preparation**
    - Cook the bacon on a skillet
    - Remove the bacon from the pan and set aside
    - Throw the Brussels sprouts to the pan and cook them in the bacon grease over medium to low for about 10-15 minutes until brown and soft. Keep stirring every few minutes.
    - Cut the bacon strips into smaller pieces.
    - Add the bacon strips and seasoning to the Brussels sprouts.
    - Stir fry and enjoy!

Approximate calories: 450 (30g protein/35g fat/6g carbs)

Pan Fried Avocado

If you don't have a lot of time or aren't that hungry, you can easily have a simple yet tasty small little meal.

- **Ingredients**
    - 1 avocado
    - 2 tablespoons of butter, coconut oil or lard
    - Sea salt
- **Preparation**
    - Cut avocado in half and remove the pit.
    - Peel and cut into small cubes.
    - Melt the butter over medium heat.
    - Add the avocado and cook for a few minutes until only slightly brown. Stir occasionally. Don't overdo with the heat, as fats will go rancid.
    - Season with salt and *voila!*

Approximate calories: 450 (5g protein/40g fat/10g carbs)

The alternative would be to simply eat the avocado raw, still add some salt and coat it with olive oil or cold butter instead. Tastes amazing!

Breakfast Tacos

A great Mexican recipe for about 2-4 tacos.

- **Ingredients**
    - 1 cup of Mozzarella cheese, shredded
    - 6 large eggs
    - 2 tablespoons of butter

- 3 bacon strips
- ½ avocado
- Salt and pepper
- ½ cup of cheddar cheese

- **Preparation**
    - Cook the bacon in the oven for about 15-20 minutes at 375 F/190 C.
    - Heat the Mozzarella cheese, about 1/3 cup at a time, on a pan on medium heat. Shape them like the shells of a taco.
    - Let the cheese get brownish on the edges, which takes about 2-3 minutes.
    - Use a pair of tongs to lift the shell up from the pan and drape it over a wooden spoon resting on a pot. Let them hang there.
    - Scramble the eggs in butter and stir occasionally until done. Season with salt and pepper.
    - Take a spoon and add a third of your scrambled eggs, avocado and bacon into each taco shell.
    - Sprinkle cheddar cheese over your tacos.
    - Just like the real stuff.

Approximate calories for the whole batch: 1300-1400 (120g protein/110g fat/5g carbs)

Approximate calories for 1 taco: 350 (30g protein/30g fat/2g carbs)

Coconut Keto Cereal

If you've ever been a child (...), then you probably downed a lot of breakfast cereal. Tony the Tiger said its *"Grrreat!"* and our parents believed them. It has a lot of essential vitamins and minerals – everything a growing organism needs. But they're also filled with sugar, syrup, grains which make them not so great after all.

Yet again, we don't have to give up our crunchy cereal in the morning and can still eat keto. This recipe cooks the cereal in bulk. The actual serving size depends on how much you're going to eat.

- **Ingredients**
    - 1 whole package of coconut flakes
    - Cinnamon
    - Stevia (optional)
    - Unsweetened almond milk
    - A few strawberries or blueberries
    - A handful of mixed nuts
    - 1 teaspoon of coconut oil
- **Preparation**
    - Preheat the oven to 350 F/180 C.
    - Grease a baking pan with coconut oil or use baking parchment instead.
    - Pour the coconut flakes on the pan and cook them for about 5 minutes. Keep watch the whole time.
    - Shuffle the flakes and stir them around. Keep cooking until they're slightly tan and toasted.
    - Take the flakes out and sprinkle with cinnamon.

- To eat, take about ½ cups of the chips and put them into a bowl. Pour in the almond milk, slice in the berries and add a few more nuts.
- Bon appetite!

Approximate calories for 1 cup of cereal with 1 cup of almond milk: 500 (6g protein/50g fat/6g carbs).

Bacon Bread

By now, it's starting to resemble a conspiracy. Yes, a bacon conspiracy. Who can get sick of bacon? Nobody, I'm telling you, that umami taste is created by the gods. This is going to be the last bacon recipe, I promise.

- **Ingredients**
    - 1 package of bacon
- **Preparation**
    - Preheat the oven to 400 F/200 C.
    - Cut the bacon strips in half.
    - Set up a baking pan with tinfoil or parchment paper.
    - Use 4-6 bacon slices and weave them together to create bread tops.

- Cook them in the oven for 20 minutes until crispy
- Take the pan out of the oven and use a spatula to remove the bacon bread.
- Use paper towels to pat them down and allow them to cool for a few minutes.

- Eat them by themselves or add some additional toppings like a real sandwich.

Approximate calories per 1 slice of bacon bread: 350 (25g protein/30g fat/0g carbs).

One thing you have to be mindful of is that bacon doesn't replace quality nutrition. There are other foods that have a lot more health benefits, such as fish, eggs and vegetables. You can eat bacon but don't make it the end-all be-all of your meals. Seafood is a lot richer in nutrients.

Cauli Hash

- **Ingredients**

- 2 tablespoons of butter or ghee
- ½ onion, chopped
- 2-4 garlic cloves, minced
- About 1 pound of cauliflower steamed and chopped into small chunks.
- Turmeric, ginger, salt and pepper
- ½ green bell peppers

- **Preparation**
  - Sautee the onions in butter for a few minutes over medium heat.
  - After 5 minutes, add the garlic and bell pepper
  - Squeeze all excess water from your steamed cauliflower. Add it to the pan and sautee for 5-10 minutes until brown and crispy.
  - Add the seasoning and toss all of the ingredients around for another 2 minutes.
  - Throw the mix into a bowl and have a nice meal!

Approximate calories: 350 (12g protein/25g fat/12g carbs).

Avocado Mayonnaise

Now, you would also like some tasty dipping with those chips, am I right? Thought so. Ketchup and other sauces are out of the question for obvious reasons.

The problem with regular mayonnaise is that it's filled with added sugar and trans fats which is the worst possible combination. It spikes our insulin and causes inflammation. That's something we should try to avoid as much as possible. Luckily, we can have something as tasty without having to put in a lot of effort. By simply replacing some of the ingredients we can have a sauce that's healthy and cheap.

- **Ingredients:**
    - 2-4 Egg yolks
    - 200 ml of Olive oil
    - 1 whole lemon
    - 1 avocado
    - 1 teaspoon of mustard seeds
    - Tabasco sauce
    - 4-5 garlic cloves
    - Salt and pepper
- **Preparation:**
    - Separate the yolks and cut open the avocado.
    - Put them together into a jar and mix vigorously or use a blender.

- Add the seasoning and squeeze in the lemon juice.

- Crush the garlic cloves and mustard seeds and throw them in as well.

- A few drops of Tabasco for the extra burn.

- Slowly pour in the olive oil and keep mixing. Do it steadily and maintain a constant stream.

- Once it starts to thicken you know it's done.

- For more texture add more avocados or peanut butter.

- For more liquid add more oil or yolks.

Approximate calories per tablespoon: 100 (2g protein/9g fat/1g carbs).

The best way to make it is in bulk. Grab a jar and make a lot of it in advance. Store it in the freezer and use it as a sauce on your dishes. It tastes even better than the conventional mayonnaise and is completely keto-proof.

Beef Stroganoff

A simple delicious dish you can use to get in the necessary creatine from red meat.

- **Ingredients**
    - 1 tablespoon of butter
    - 1 medium onion, chopped
    - 2 to 3 garlic cloves, chopped
    - 1 pound of grass-fed ground beef
    - 1 tablespoons of heavy cream
    - Salt and pepper
    - 2 cups of spinach or other green vegetable
- **Preparation**

- Add the butter to a heated cast iron pan over medium to high heat.
- Once it's melted, add the onions and garlic. Cook until soft, for about 5 minutes.
- Add the beef and cook until desired doneness.
- Reduce the heat to low and add the cheese on top, letting it melt gently.
- Add the cream, seasoning and stir well. Let it sit for a few minutes with the heat turned off.
- Either cook the spinach inside the same mixture or use it as a bedding for the meat. Both options work and taste great.
- Enjoy!

Approximate calories: 1200-1400 (100g protein/100g fat/10g carbs)

Keto Spaghetti Squash

Another Italian classic that doesn't require wheat or whole grains.

- **Ingredients**
    - 1 spaghetti squash
    - 2 tablespoons of butter
    - 1/4 cup of heavy cream or coconut milk
    - Salt and pepper
    - ½ cups of grated cheese
    - A pinch of basil
- **Preparation**
    - Preheat the oven to 375 F/180 C
    - Slice the squash in half, lengthwise, and remove the seeds and pulp.
    - Wrap both halves in aluminum foil, place them face-up on a baking sheet and bake for about 30-40 minutes.

- Once done, scoop out the flesh with a fork, which will create these spaghetti like figures.

- Melt the butter over medium heat and add the heavy cream, salt, cheese and basil. Cook for about 10-15 minutes at a light simmer, while stirring every once in a while.
- Add the spaghetti squash, mix and enjoy!

Approximate calories: 400 (8g protein/30g fat/15g carbs)

Cheesy Grated Cauliflower

Like with bacon, you rarely get sick of cauliflower. It's the most versatile food at our disposal that can be used for numerous dishes, including by itself.

- **Ingredients**
    - 1 large head of cauliflower
    - 1 1/2 cups of shredded cheese
    - 1/2 cup of heavy cream
    - ¼ teaspoon of black pepper
    - ½ teaspoon of sea salt
- **Preparation**
    - Preheat the oven to 400F/200C.
    - Chop the cauliflower into bite-sized pieces and put them in a steamer pot. Bring the water to boil and let it simmer on low to medium heat.
    - Steam the cauliflower for 10-15 minutes or until it's tender enough to be pierced with a fork.

- Mix the cheese and heavy cream in a baking dish. Stir in seasoning and let it simmer.
- Add the cauliflower to the cheese mixture and stir around until it's well coated.
- Bake for about 30 minutes or until the top is nicely brown.
- Remove from the oven and let it sit for 5-10 minutes to allow the sauce to thicken just a bit.
- Enjoy!

Approximate calories for the entire batch: 800(50g protein/60g fat/15g carbs)

Keto Sushi

Despite the oriental origin of rice, you can even have sushi on keto. It's great and tastes amazing. This recipe is about 10-20 servings, depending on how wide you'll cut the sheets.

- **Ingredients**
    - 1 cup of cauliflower
    - 6oz/150g cream cheese
    - 1-2 tablespoon of rice vinegar (unseasoned)
    - 5 sheets of Nori
    - 1 large cucumber
    - ½ avocado
    - 5oz/150g salmon
- **Preparation**
    - Use a food processor to "rice" the cauliflower into rice-sized pieces.
    - Slice the cucumber on each end, and slice off each side as well.
    - Cook the cauliflower rice on a hot pan and let it simmer for just a bit.

- Dry out the cauliflower, add it to a bowl with cream cheese and rice vinegar. Mix together and put it into the freezer.
- Slice the avocado into small strips and take out the seed.
- Lay down the nori sheet on a bamboo roller. Spread the cauliflower mix on top, leaving about ¾ inches of space at the top. This is the thinner layer.
- Place all of the filling items into the sushi roll and roll it tightly.
- いただきます (itadakimasu) – Bon Appetite in Japanese.

Approximate calories for the entire recipe: 800 (55g protein/55g protein/15g carbs).

Approximate calories for 1 piece of sushi: 45 (3g protein/4g fat/1g carbs).

Coconut Milk Ice Cream

Despite the lack of sugar in the diet it doesn't mean that we can't be having something sweet. To be honest, the umami taste of bacon feels like candy. Maybe it's just me. We can still have ice cream and bake cakes using keto friendly ingredients and they're even better. This recipe is completely dairy free and suitable for everyone.

- **Ingredients:**
    - 2 cups of coconut milk
    - 2 eggs
    - 2 tablespoons of butter and olive oil
    - 1 teaspoon of vanilla extract or Stevia (optional)
    - Nuts according to preference.
    - 1 tablespoon of coconut flakes

- ½ cups of blueberries
- 1 teaspoon of cinnamon

- **Preparation:**

    - Separate the egg yolks and whites.

    - Whip the whites until they turn soft.

    - Mix vigorously or blend together butter, olive oil, seasoning while simultaneously adding in the yolks. Do it one by one and slowly until a smooth mixture forms.

    - Pour in the coconut milk and slowly add the egg whites.

    - Keep mixing it all together to make it more fluffy.

    - It should begin to become thicker after a while. For texture add more eggs.

    - Throw in the nuts, blueberries, coconut flakes and cinnamon.

- You can put it in the freezer for a few hours for it to turn more solid or eat right away. The perfect dessert for a hot day.

Approximate calories: 500 (20g protein/40g fat/5g carbs).

Keto Pancakes

Everyone's childhood is probably filled with memories about having pancakes on Sunday. They're great but not for our health because of the gluten and high-fat-carb combo. Fortunately, there is another solution – the keto way. By replacing some of the ingredients, we can still enjoy a healthy tasty dessert.

- **Ingredients:**
    - 2-3 eggs
    - 2 cups of coconut milk or heavy cream (has twice the calories)
    - 2 tablespoons of butter or coconut oil
    - 2oz/50g of almond or coconut flour
    - 1 teaspoon of cinnamon
    - 1/3 cup of blueberries and coconut flakes
- **Preparation:**
    - Beat the eggs until soft.
    - Pour in cream and flour according to preference and texture.
    - Mix them together with cinnamon.

- Heat the pan with butter.

- Pour in the pancake mixture and cook on both sides.

- While in the pan throw some coconut flakes on top.

- Serve on a plate with blueberries.

This recipe doesn't even have to involve flour. We can get the same results by using only eggs and cream. It won't look like batter but there hardly is any other difference.

Approximate calories for 3 pancakes: 650 (40g protein/50g fat/6g carbs).

Keto Chocolate

You can eat dark chocolate on keto and it's incredibly healthy for your health. What's more, it tastes a lot better than the regular milk chocolate equivalent.

You can put only 1 small piece of 80%+ chocolate that's darker than night and be incredibly satiated. Your taste buds will light up but won't cause any additional cravings.

Good quality dark chocolate can be hard to come by. No worries, you can make your own with.

- **Ingredients**
    - 2 tablespoons of coconut oil
    - 2 tablespoons of raw cacao butter
    - 3 tablespoons of cacao powder
    - 1 cup of coconut milk or almond milk (optional, if you want a milkier texture)
    - 1 teaspoon of vanilla extract
    - 1 teaspoon of cinnamon
    - A pinch of sea salt

- 1 teaspoon of Stevia

- **Preparation**
    - Melt the coconut oil and cacao butter in a skillet over very low heat. Let the texture get softer slowly. Don't make it boil.
    - Once the mixture is melted, turn off the heat and mix in the cacao powder. It should look dark and creamy.
    - If you want more of a milky taste, mix in the coconut milk.
    - Stir in the cinnamon, salt, stevia and the vanilla extract.
    - Allow the chocolate mixture to cool until it reaches room temperature.
    - Put the mixture in the refrigerator for 30 minutes until it becomes solid.
    - After the chocolate has solidified, break it apart and put it in a glass container.
    - Savor the taste by eating small pieces at a time.

Approximate calories for the entire batch: 500 (5g protein/45g carbs/3g carbs).

Chocolate Peanut Butter Fat Bomb Cups

Another incredible fat bomb at our disposal for nuclear taste bombs.

- **Ingredients**
    - 2 tablespoons of coconut oil
    - 2 tablespoons of cacao powder
    - 3 tablespoons of sunflower seeds or hemp seeds
    - 1/4 cup of heavy cream
    - 1 teaspoon of vanilla extract
    - 1 teaspoon of Stevia
    - ¼ cup of shredded coconut flakes

- 1 teaspoon of cinnamon
- **Preparation**
    - Mix the dry ingredients together with the coconut oil. It should turn into a paste.
    - Add heavy cream and the seasoning. Stir once more.
    - Lay out the shredded coconut flakes on to a plate.
    - Use your hands to roll out balls from the paste and then roll them in the coconut flakes.
    - Lay the fat bombs onto a tray and set in the freezer for about 20 minutes.
    - Rejoice!

Approximate calories for 5 bombs: 900 (12g protein/85g fat/6g carbs).

Approximate calories per bomb: 180 (3g protein/17g fat/1g carbs).

Vanilla Ice Cream

Another easy to make ice cream. This time it's the classical vanilla taste.

- **Ingredients**
    - 1/2 cup of heavy cream (more calories) or 1 cup of coconut milk
    - 1 teaspoon of Stevia (optional)
    - 1 teaspoon of vanilla extract
    - 3 cups of ice
    - 4 teaspoons of sea salt
- **Preparation**
    - Pour the heavy cream, stevia and vanilla extract into a small airtight plastic bag and shake.
    - Put the ice and salt in an airtight container.
    - Lay the plastic bag on top of the ice and close the container. Shake it vigorously for about 2 minutes.

- o Remove the plastic bag from the container and wash off the excess salt.
- o Pout the ice cream out of the bag into a bowl.
- o Serve immediately.

Approximate calories for ice cream with heavy cream: 420 (3g protein/44g fat/2g carbs).

Approximate calories for coconut milk: 400 (3g protein/40g fat/1g carbs).

Keto Brownies

Okay...now we're getting almost out of hand. How ridiculous does it sound that you can also bake brownies and cakes on keto. The myth of refined wheat flour can be laid aside. Time for much healthier options to take its place in the kitchen

- **Ingredients**
    - 1 cup of Golden Flaxseed Meal
    - ¼ cup of cacao powder
    - 1 tablespoon of cinnamon
    - ½ tablespoons of baking powder
    - ½ teaspoons of salt
    - 1 large egg
    - 2 tablespoons of coconut oil
    - ½ cup of pumpkin puree
    - 1 teaspoon of vanilla extract
    - ¼ cups of almond flakes
- **Preparation**
    - Preheat the oven to 350F/175C. Combine all of the ingredients in a deep mixing bowl and mix to combine
    - Take out a muffin tin and spoon about ¼ cup of batter into each muffin liner.
    - Sprinkle almond flakes over the muffins.

- Bake in the oven for about 15 minutes. Once the muffins begin to rise and set on top, they're ready.
- Enjoy!

Approximate calories for the entire batch: 1000 (55g protein/80g fat/10g carbs).

Approximate calories for 1 brownie: 150 (9g protein/13g fat/2g carbs).

Just a few examples. It's simple keto.

Don't take the easy way out and buy prepackaged meals or TV dinners. Take the time to cook your own food and enjoy it.

Make it into a fun family activity. That's what the ketogenic lifestyle is also about.

How Should You Eat?

This also raises the question of how you should structure your eating plan. To be honest, it all comes down to personal preference. Your lifestyle and habits are completely different from mine. It depends on your goals and current condition as well. I can only give you some practical tips form my own experience.

On the ketogenic diet you don't get as hungry as you would on a medium to high carbohydrate one. For me, this is a blessing because I don't like to spend time eating that frequently. Don't get me wrong – I'm a total foodie. But the benefits of intermittent fasting are too good for me to pass on them. You don't have to eat any more than twice a day. At least that's what I do.

Snacking isn't a good habit to have, even on keto. It's probably one of the biggest reasons why people can't seem to lose weight. Because of their mindless eating, they won't even notice how many calories they've actually consumed and won't get psychologically satisfied either.

Whatever the case might be, you shouldn't eat more than 3 meals a day. It's best to implement some intermittent fasting strategies into your daily schedule, which is a whole nother topic. If you want to know more about this, then check out my blog listed at the end of this book.

When in ketosis you reduce muscle catabolism to a bare minimum and won't have to eat as often. Trust me, looking at my experience and body composition, it's safe to say I know what I'm talking about. Your metabolism won't crash and burn if you skip breakfast. I'm actually feeling stronger and mentally sharper while fasting. You just need to teach your body how to burn its own fat for fuel.

Me personally, I have only 2 meals a day. Some of that fatty egg yolk beverage, which also call under a different name - Empowered Superhero Coffee, at noon keeps me satiated for the entire day. At dinner I have some delicious low carb meal, such as pork chops or salmon with butter roasted vegetables.

On keto it's simple. The foods eaten are so tasty that you rarely get sick of them. This makes it a very sustainable diet to follow for both weight loss and maintaining a lean physique as well. Who gets sick of bacon and eggs? Nobody, I'm telling you. It's like a conspiracy theory. That umami taste is created by the Gods.

Chapter VIII
Simple Keto Supplements

Despite our access to abundant contemporary food we're still missing some key ingredients - the micronutrients. To overcome this flaw there are some supplements we should be taking.

Health is not something to be taken for granted and being superhuman requires doing what's necessary for achieving that status. What matters more about any type of food is not its caloric proportions but the minerals, enzymes, vitamins etc. and what hormonal effect it has on the organism.

With the industrialization of food all of that has suffered. Our soils are being depleted from their vital life force with the use of fertilizers, spraying of toxic fumes, usage of GMOs, radiation, travel pollution and many other things. All for the purpose of creating more empty calories and food without any actually beneficial content.

A word of caution. There are a lot of supplements we could be taking. However, that doesn't mean we should start gorging on piles of tablets and numerous pills. It's not about becoming a substance junkie, but a self-empowered being who simply covers all of the necessary micronutrients through the usage of natural yet still manufactured additives.

We don't need to take a whole lot, simply some which everyone needs and especially those that we're individually most deficient of. That's something we have to find out ourselves.

We don't need to fear these pharmaceuticals just because their artificial form. They are just natural ingredients that have been processed and put into a bottle or a powder.

All of the supplements that I have listed here are least processed and free from any additional garbage, such as preservatives, GMO, gluten, starch, sugar etc. They're keto-proof and friendly.

Additionally, we should always try to stick to real whole foods as much as possible. Supplements are just that - supplementation for some of the deficiencies we fail to get from what we actually eat. They're not magical but simply give us the extra edge.

The effects these products have can be derived from natural foods as well. In the form of a pill or a powder they're simply microscopic and packaged nutrition. Taking them will grant us access to optimal health - the utmost level of wellbeing and performance both physical and mental.

In this list are all of the supplements I am personally taking because of their importance, as well as the additional benefits we get. However, I do not advise anyone to take any of them unless they are aware of their medical condition and don't know about the possible side effects or issues that may or may not follow.

Before taking anything we ought to educate ourselves about the topic and consult a professional physician. The

responsibility is solely on the individual and I will take none.

Not Really Supplements

To start off I'm going to list the supplements we should be taking, each and every one of us, as they are something that we're definitely all deficient of and also promote Superhuman wellbeing.

Not everything we consume ought to come in the form of a pill. A lot of micronutrients can be found in unprocessed products as well, we simply need to add them to our diet and reap the benefits. They are most natural and completely free from the touch of man. Therefore, they come first and are of utmost value.

We already touched upon the health benefits of turmeric, ginger and cinnamon. You should consume them every single day. In case you missed it, here they are again.

- **Turmeric.** One of the best spices we can use is curcumin or turmeric. It has a lot of medicinal properties, such as anti-inflammatory compounds, increase of antioxidants and brain health. Also, it fights and prevents many diseases, such as Arthritis, Alzheimer's and even cancer. In addition to that, it tastes amazing and can be added to everything. I sprinkle it on all foods and run out quite quickly which is why I also buy it in bulk so that it's cheaper. You can also take a capsule.

- **Ginger.** Continuing on with turmeric's brother. It has almost as much health benefits. In addition to that, it lowers blood sugar levels, fights heart disease, treats chronic indigestion, may reduce menstrual pain for women, lowers cholesterol and heals muscle pain. Once again, bulk or capsule.

- **Cinnamon.** These three create the most important natural spices we should be eating on a daily basis. They're incredibly cheap and easy to come by yet have amazing health as well as performance enhancing benefits. Moreover, they all make food taste amazing. Cinnamon falls into the same category as ginger and turmeric - superfoods, because it truly empowers us. In addition to the same medicinal properties it also increases insulin sensitivity, fights neurodegenerative disease and bacterial infections. What's best about it is that it can be added to not only salty foods but on desserts as well. I even add it to my coffee. The best to use is Ceylon or „true" cinnamon.

- **Green tea.** It isn't an actual supplement but is still extremely empowering. In fact, it can be considered to be the healthiest beverage of the world after water. It improves health, brain function, fat oxidation and detoxifies the system. Additionally, lowers blood pressure and prevents all types of disease, including Alzheimer's and cancer. We don't need to take pills with extracts but can get all of the benefits by simply drinking a cup a day. However, to get all of the benefits we need to be consuming about 15-30 cups. Using a capsule would be very efficient.

- **Garlic.** It has a strong taste and smell but is incredibly healthy nonetheless. Chopping garlic cloves forms a compound called allicin, which, once digested, travels all over the body and exerts its potent biological effects. It fights all illness, especially the cold, reduces blood pressure, improves cholesterol levels, contains antioxidants, increases longevity, detoxifies the body from metals, promotes bone health and is delicious. Because of its flavor it makes a great addition to meals. It also comes in capsuled form.

Supplements you HAVE to Take

Moving on with actual supplements. These things we're all deficient of and they also take our performance to the next level, they empower us.

- **Fish/Krill oil.** It's rich in omega-3 fatty acids, which are great for the brain and heart. The counterpart to that is omega-6, which are pro-inflammatory and bad for us. Omega-6 can be found in a lot of processed foods and vegetable oils, which we would want to avoid anyway. For our body to be healthy the omega-3's need to be in balance with the omega-6's. Unfortunately, that balance can be easily tipped off as every amount of omega-6 requires triple the amount of omega-3 to reduce the negative effects. Additionally, fish oil has DHA, which promotes brain functioning, fights inflammation, supports bone health, increases physical performance etc. Naturally, it can be found in fatty fish such as salmon, herring, mackerel and sardines. Fish oil falls into the same category because of its vital importance for superhuman health. It can be used easily as a capsule or liquidized. Taking one teaspoon a day will drastically improve your life. Krill oil might simply be a more potent and bioavailable source. Make sure to use wild caught sources to avoid mercury poisoning.

- **Vitamin D-3.** This is the sunshine vitamin and is one of the most important nutrients. Life exists on Earth because of the Sun. D-3 governs almost every function within us starting from DNA repair and metabolic processes making it a foundation to everything that goes on. It's embedded in nutritious food, given it has received enough exposure to solar light. Vitamin D-3 fights cardiovascular, autoimmune and infective diseases. Of course, the best source would be to get it from the Sun but that is not always possible because of seasonality and location. It can be consumed as oil or a capsule.

- **Magnesium.** Another foundational mineral. It comprises 99% of the body's mineral content and governs almost all of the processes. Magnesium helps to build bones, enables nerves to function and is essential for the production of energy from food. This is especially beneficial for the physically active. Some people who are depressed get headaches because of this deficiency. Because our soils are quite depleted magnesium needs to be supplemented. It can also be used as an oil on your skin for greater absorption in specific areas.

Supplements Empowered

We have covered all of the supplements we should be taking no matter what, the most important and essential ones. Now I'll get down to the empowering ones.

They are not foundational but beneficial nonetheless. With the help of these we can transcend the boundary between healthy and superhuman performance as they will take us to the next level.

- **Creatine Monohydrate.** Creatine is an organic acid produced in the liver that helps to supply energy to cells all over the body, especially muscles. It enhances ATP production and allows for muscle fibers to contract faster, quicker, and makes them overall stronger. That means increased physical performance with explosive and strength based movements and sprinting. However, it doesn't end there. Creatine has been found to improve cognitive functioning, as it's a nootropic as well, improving mental acuity and memory. Naturally, it can be found most in red meat. It's [dirty cheap](#) and easy to consume, as only 5 grams per day will do wonders and doing so won't make a person big nor bulky.

- **Pro- and prebiotics.** Having a well working digestive system is incredibly vital for getting the most nutrients out of our food. Industrialization has done another disservice to us by destroying all of the bacteria in the food we consume, the good and the bad, and replacing them with preservatives. We might be eating but we're not actually deriving a lot of nutrients. In order to have a healthy gut we need to have a well-functioning microbiome. Naturally, food is full of living organisms. Sauerkraut, raw milk, yoghurt, unprocessed meat all have good bacteria in them. With there being no life in our food, we need to create it within us ourselves. Probiotics are alive microorganisms in a pill that transport these good bacteria into our gut for improved digestion and immune system. Prebiotics are different, they're not alive, but plant fiber that feeds the bacteria. They're indigestible parts of the vegetable that go through our digestive track into our gut where the bacteria then eat them. If you don't like eating a lot of broccoli and spinach, then you should still get a lot of fiber into your diet.

- **Thyroid supplementation.** The thyroid gland is incredibly important for our health because it regulates the functioning of our metabolism. Moreover, because of its location in our throat it also is a connective point between the brain and the rest of the body. This organ is a part of an incredibly complex system which creates this intertwined relationship between the two. With a low functioning thyroid one will have an impeded metabolism, suffer hypothyroidism and many other diseases because of the necessary hormones will not be produced. Promoting thyroid functioning can be done by taking [iodine supplementation](#) or eating a lot of [sea vegetables](#). The daily requirements for selenium can be met with eating only 2-3 [Brazil nuts](#).

- **Multivitamin.** There are definitely a lot of vitamins to be covered for our body to not only be healthy but function at its peak. It would be unreasonable to take too many tablets or pills while neglecting the importance of real food. However, taking a multivitamin that has a lot of beneficial minerals all combined into one [bottle](#) is very effective and will most definitely be useful.

- **Maca.** Another superfood comes from the Peruvian mountains and is the root of ginseng. It has numerous amounts of vitamins and minerals in it, such as magnesium zinc, copper etc. Also, it promotes hormone functioning for both men and women, as well as increases our energy production just like creatine does. It can either be powdered or made into a tablet.

- **GABA.** Called gamma-aminobutyric acid, it's the main inhibitory neurotransmitter, and regulates the nerve impulses in the human body. Therefore, it is important for both physical and mental performance, as both of them are connected to the nervous system. Also, GABA is to an extent responsible for causing relaxation and calmness, helping to produce BDNF.

- **Chaga mushroom.** Chaga is a mushroom that grows on birch trees. It's extremely beneficial for supporting the immune system, has anti-oxidative and soothing properties, lowers blood pressure and cholesterol. Also, consuming it will promote the health and integrity of the adrenal glands. This powder can be added to teas or other warm beverages. Or you can grind it yourself.

- **MCT oil.** For nutritional ketosis having an additional source of ketone bodies will be beneficial. MCT stands for medium chain triglycerides which are fat molecules that can be digested more rapidly than normal fat ones, which are usually long chain triglycerides. Doing so will enable the brain to have immediate access to abundant energy and a deeper state of ketosis. Basically, it's glucose riding the vessel of ketones. Naturally, it's extracted from coconut oil and is an enhanced liquidized version of it. Additionally, I also eat raw coconut flakes, which have MCTs in them.

- **Collagen protein.** Collagen provides the fastest possible healthy tissue repair, bone renewal and recovery after exercise. It can also boost mental clarity, reduce inflammation, clear your skin, promote joint integrity, reduces aging and builds muscle. Naturally, it's found in tendons and ligaments, that can be consumed by eating meat. As a supplement it can be used as protein powder or as gelatin capsules.

This is the list of supplements we should be taking. It includes the most important ones, the essential, which we should be taking no matter what, as well as the not so vital that simply make us more empowered and give us the extra edge. Nothing replaces good food, but proper and educated supplementation will fix some of the loopholes.

Bonus Chapter

How to Get into Ketosis Super Fast

Before you start living the ketogenic lifestyle, you may want to speed up your adaptation process. This chapter teaches you how to get into nutritional ketosis super fast.

To get into ketosis we have to either:

- Fast for a prolonged amount of time.

- Restrict our carbohydrate intake to a bare minimum.

Both options are very effective ways of inducing ketosis.

However, those two things aren't always enough. **Someone who is burning sugar may not ever be able to get into ketosis, despite following the guidelines.** The body is just too addicted to sugar and enters an energy crisis.

To provide energy for the brain and body, it is necessary to have a substitute for glucose. If you want to become fat adapted, then you have to promote the production of ketone bodies as well. To do that, we would have to consume fat that is easily absorbed and gives quick energy.

The #1 source of quality fat is probably MCT oil. There are also exogenous ketones but at the moment they are not that commercially available. For habitual use, MCTs get the job done and are great.

To promote ketone production, we can eat any other type of fat as well. Coconut oil, grass-fed butter, ghee and olive oil are only slightly less effective.

How to Get Into Ketosis Fast.

Fasting is the most natural and effective ways of inducing ketosis. After a few days the body will be utilizing primarily fat for fuel because there is no glucose left to be found. In addition to that, it will derive energy solely from the adipose tissue.

To not become excessively gluconeogenic and begin to cannibalize your precious muscles and organs, then you need to provide yourself with at least some form of energy.

Consuming only fat, with no other macronutrient will not even put you into a fed state. The calories will not cross the blood-brain barrier and it actually mimicks fasting. Because your blood sugar levels will not be affected, you will continue to fast. The exception is that now you will have higher ketone levels and increased energy.

This is called fat fasting. It takes the 2 best ways of getting into ketosis and makes the adaptation process even faster.

Doing this will not be very taxing to the body. For a sugar burner it will definitely be quite difficult. Lowering their carbohydrate intake even just a little bit will cause withdrawal symptoms. What would you expect from a full on ban then?

For someone who already knows how to use fat for fuel, this will be actually quite enjoyable. It will feel like fasting but you'll have a lot of energy. After a few days, you should be in quite deep ketosis.

But how much fat should you consume? There isn't any upper or lower limit, really. However, there will definitely be a point of diminishing returns. Once that threshold has been crossed, you won't get any extra benefit from consuming more MCTs. You'll simply be eating calories.

It's better to keep your fat intake as low as possible and use it only when necessary. To not exit your fasted state, you would only want to take one teaspoon a few times a day. This would total under 500 calories that are all derived from fat.

Mistakes to Avoid

Fat fasting is a great way to get into ketosis faster, but it shouldn't be taken too far. During the adaptation phase, you'll be still quite catabolic and dependent of glucose.

You're still going to have to go through several days of adaptation before you make a complete shift. But you don't want to be fasting for that long.

If you're obese or sedentary, then you can get away with it easily. If you're physically active and a fit individual, then you shouldn't fast for that long. In that case, you would want to do it for a day or two on days when you're not training. This should only be a strategy to kick-start the process.

Also, you wouldn't want to neglect the principles of ketogenic dieting. This is not a quick fix, but simply a very time-efficient strategy. Don't think that this will put you into deep ketosis for the rest of your life. After breaking the fast you would still want to continue eating low carb, to stay adapted.

Conclusion
Beyond Burning Fat and Ketosis

This is it! You're well on your way towards becoming a much stronger, healthier, smarter and happier version of yourself. Simple Keto gives you all the information you need to start eating the ketogenic diet and living the lifestyle.

If you're like me, then you don't like taking health for granted. It's our most valuable asset, as it influences the overall quality of our life. That's why I prefer eating low carb. For me, it's not about weight loss but for the well-being it gives me. The same can happen for you.

Ketosis is an extremely efficient weapon against obesity and diabetes. Its effect doesn't lie in the actual mMols or blood sugar levels but in the suppression of insulin and carbohydrate restriction. That's why I think we don't need to nor should be ketogenic all of the time. We're already in mild ketosis after an overnight fast and eating low carb the rest of the day is an easy way to increase your longevity and health.

Once you become fat adapted, you've created these essential ketogenic pathways within your own biology and will know how to utilize ketones as fuel. The initial period is necessary for these mechanisms to occur. Afterwards you can still eat keto but don't have to worry about whether or not you're in the right range. You'll know it once you hit the sweet spot.

That's why I'm going to share with you a concept of mine called optimal nutrition. It can be grasped under a single sentence, which goes as follows:

Optimal nutrition is eating the right things, in the right amounts at the right time.

I do not know about you but I think there cannot be made a better definition than that. It covers all of what we need to know OBJECTIVELY, meaning that it is not taken out of context and can be applied to any situation. We simply need to decipher it and make it fit our demands.

Keto is a part of that, but it may not fit into the paradigm of optimal nutrition all of the time. For the most part it does. Even

I, who trains quite hard and often, feel this way. My body is very insulin sensitive but I still prefer to use fat for fuel.

On this note I'm going to end the book. Simple keto, right?

Ultimate Keto Meal Plan

I've also created a 21 day ketogenic meal plan called Ultimate Keto, which will put ultimately into ketosis. It will help you to start a well-formulated ketogenic diet as a long term thing. Check it out.

Get Your 21-Day Meal Plan at
http://www.siimland.com/ultimate-keto-meal-plan/

More Books from the Author

Read more books in my Simple Keto series. They're more advanced protocols of the ketogenic diet and used to maximize athletic performance while eating low carb.

Find out how to workout on keto and build muscle from the book Keto Bodybuilding

Keto Bodybuilding: Build Lean Muscle and Burn Fat at the Same Time by Eating a Low Carb Ketogenic Bodybuilding Diet and Get the Physique of a Greek God

Keto Cycle the Cyclical Ketogenic Diet Book

Target Keto the Targeted Ketogenic Diet Book

Vegan Keto: the Vegan Ketogenic Diet

Optimal Nutrition Program: Eat to Become Superhuman

Intermittent Fasting and Feasting: Use Strategic Periods of Undereating and Overfeeding to Unleash the Most Powerful Anabolic Hormones of Your Body

Also, other books of mine.

Becoming a Self Empowered Being

Leave a Review on Amazon!

If you liked this book, then I would appreciate it, if you could leave a 5-star review on Amazon. It helps me out a ton and is the least you can do to help other people start a ketogenic diet as well.

About the Author.

Hello, my name is Siim Land and I'm a holistic health practitioner, a fitness expert, an author and a self-empowered being. Ever since my childhood I've been engaged with personal development and self-actualization. As a kid, I made the decision of improving the state of mankind and transcending humanity towards the better. My journey has lead me on an Odyssey of body-mind-spirit, during which I've managed to develop and enhance every aspect of my being. My philosophy is based around achieving self-mastery and excellence first and foremost. What comes after that is the mission of empowering others to do the same. That's what I've dedicated my life to and am doing daily. To do that, I'm always trying to improve upon my own physiology, psychology and biology. I dream of a better world, in which mankind isn't separated from one another and is working towards reaching their truest potential.

Contact me at my blog: http://siimland.com/contact

References

Links to academic articles and research studies. If you're on the paperback version, then you can simply Google them and you'll find them right away.

---

[i] Body composition and hormonal responses to a carbohydrate-restricted diet.
[ii] A high-fat, ketogenic diet induces a unique metabolic state in mice.
[iii] What is an Essential Nutrient?
[iv] Endocrine Notes on Glucose Metabolism (PDF)
[v] Glycerol gluconeogenesis in fasting humans
[vi] Low-carbohydrate nutrition and metabolism
[vii] The Expensive-Tissue Hypothesis: The Brain and the Digestive System in Human and Primate Evolution
[viii] The Effects of a Ketogenic Diet on Exercise Metabolism and Physical Performance in Off-Road Cyclists
[ix] Nonenzymatic glucosylation and glucose-dependent cross-linking of protein.
[x] The AGE-receptor in the pathogenesis of diabetic complications.
[xi] Advanced glycation end products Key Players in Skin Aging?
[xii] The effects of a low-carbohydrate ketogenic diet and a low-fat diet on mood, hunger, and other self-reported symptoms
[xiii] The National Cholesterol Education Program Diet vs a Diet Lower in Carbohydrates and Higher in Protein and Monounsaturated Fat
[xiv] HDL-subpopulation patterns in response to reductions in dietary total and saturated fat intakes in healthy subjects
[xv] Short-term effects of severe dietary carbohydrate-restriction advice in Type 2 diabetes--a randomized controlled trial.
[xvi] A low-carbohydrate, ketogenic diet to treat type 2 diabetes
[xvii] Metabolic syndrome and low-carbohydrate ketogenic diets in the medical school biochemistry curriculum.
[xviii] Metabolic characteristics of keto-adapted ultra-endurance runners
[xix] Ketogenic diet does not affect strength performance in elite artistic gymnasts
[xx] Nutrition and Physical Degeneration
[xxi] Liver and kidney metabolism during prolonged starvation
[xxii] Short-term fasting induces profound neuronal autophagy

[xxiii] Enhanced thermogenic response to epinephrine after 48-h starvation in humans.
[xxiv] Alternate-day fasting in nonobese subjects: effects on body weight, body composition, and energy metabolism
[xxv] Fasting enhances growth hormone secretion and amplifies the complex rhythms of growth hormone secretion in man.
[xxvi] Autophagy is required to maintain muscle mass.
[xxvii] Inflammation-Induced Alteration of Astrocyte Mitochondrial Dynamics Requires Autophagy for Mitochondrial Network Maintenance
[xxviii] Autophagy in the Pathogenesis of Disease